RM 331 .B76 2000
Brody, Howard.
The placebo response

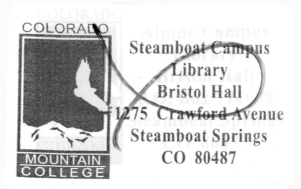

The Placebo Response

Other books by Howard Brody

The Healer's Power

Stories of Sickness

Ethical Issues in Medicine

Placebos and the Philosophy of Medicine

THE PLACEBO RESPONSE

How You Can Release The Body's Inner Pharmacy for Better Health

RECEIVED

AUG 22 2000

CMC-ALPINE CAMPUS LIBRARY

HOWARD BRODY
with Daralyn Brody

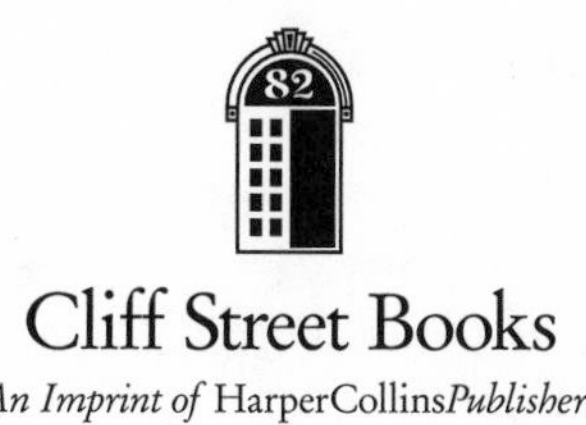

Cliff Street Books
An Imprint of HarperCollins*Publishers*

Excerpts from *Why People Don't Heal and How They Can* © 1997 by Caroline Myss, Crown Publishers, Inc., used with permission.

THE PLACEBO RESPONSE. Copyright © 2000 by Howard Brody, M.D., Ph.D. All rights reserved. Printed in the United States of America. No part of this book may be used or reproduced in any manner whatsoever without written permission except in the case of brief quotations embodied in critical articles and reviews. For information address HarperCollins Publishers Inc., 10 East 53rd Street, New York, NY 10022.

HarperCollins books may be purchased for educational, business, or sales promotional use. For information please write: Special Markets Department, HarperCollins Publishers Inc., 10 East 53rd Street, New York, NY 10022.

FIRST EDITION

Designed by Christine Weathersbee

Printed on acid-free paper

Library of Congress Cataloging-in-Publication Data has been applied for.

ISBN 0-06-019493-6

00 01 02 03 04 ❖/RRD 10 9 8 7 6 5 4 3 2 1

To Sheila and Mark
and to the many patients
who have taught us

CONTENTS

ACKNOWLEDGMENTS

In thanking those who have played an important role in the writing of this book, I must first turn to the book's co-producer, my wife, Daralyn. Daralyn has had both a direct and an indirect role. She's studied a number of types of alternative healing, and as the writing proceeded, she took charge of two special tasks. The first was to be sure that the book was evenhanded in describing both alternative and conventional medicine. The second was to organize the material with the non-scientifically trained reader in mind.

But Daralyn's influence on the book also includes her influence on my career and patterns of thinking, which, in twenty-eight years of marriage, has been considerable. Daralyn prides herself on being a right-brain person (sometimes so much so that she gives her excellent left brain too little credit). She's devoted herself to the study of the folkloric dances of Middle Eastern and Central Asian cultures. In those cultures, dance has historically been related to healing and shamanism, and this has further stimulated Daralyn's interest in the mind-body connection.

As a dancer, Daralyn tends to proceed intuitively rather than logically or verbally. Where I might ask, "Do we really understand how this works?" Daralyn might say, "If it works, does it matter?" Where I might have wanted to explain something for pages and pages, Daralyn said, "Let's get to the point—how is this useful?" For me, our relationship has been an excellent life lesson in patience and humility—two qualities, as we'll see, that help to make the physician a better partner for the patient. I think that this book is richer and deeper as a result of Daralyn's and my complementary ways of looking at the world.

A good deal of this book arises from my role as a family physician, so I next owe a deep debt of gratitude to those who taught me that craft, in medical school at the College of Human Medicine, Michigan State University, and in residency at the University of Virginia Medical Center in Charlottesville. I fear mentioning any of my valued teachers by name lest I offend someone who has been inadvertently omitted. I must, however, say a special word about the longtime chair of Family Medicine at Virginia, Dr. B. Lewis Barnett, Jr., who for many across the country has come almost to embody the ideals of family practice. It may have been in Lewis's home, sitting around his fireplace and listening to his stories drawn from twenty years of practice in a small town in South Carolina, that the connection between stories and healing first fully dawned in my mind.

I'm also grateful, of course, to my teachers in philosophy at Michigan State University, where I earned my Ph.D. and first began my scholarly inquiry into the placebo effect; and to my colleagues in the Department of Family Practice at Michigan State, who not only taught me so much over the years but who also shoulder the burden of taking care of my patients when I am out of town or otherwise unavailable.

Two of these colleagues, Drs. William C. Wadland and Janis Rygwelski, assisted me by reading an early draft of this book and commenting to me on its accuracy regarding both conventional and complementary medicine. Any mistakes that remain are purely my own.

Over the years, I have benefited from reading the writings of many experts on the placebo response, most of whom are credited in the Bibliographic Essay. Among those who have helped me through personal conversation over the years have been David Sobel, Dan Moerman, Irving Kirsch, Robert Ader, Arthur Kleinman, Robert Hahn, Ted Kaptchuk, Arthur Frank, and David Hufford. Since Dr. Howard M. Spiro and I hold what appear to be contrary views on the ethics of administering placebos, he and I have been invited to "debate" on several occasions, and I have come away from those meetings impressed with Dr. Spiro's deep, humane regard and compassion for patients and commitment to rigorous thinking.

A number of years ago, I had the privilege of participating in a project at Michigan State University known as the Center for Meaning and Health. This center was unfortunately short-lived, formally lasting only two years. Had it survived, I believe that we might have been successful through that organization in supplying a few of the missing "clues" to the nature of the placebo response, which I allude to in the following chapters—and which I am still hopeful of pursuing with some of my present colleagues. Nevertheless, I learned a great deal that went into shaping the ideas in this book from conversations with such participants as Drs. Robert Smith, Larry VanEgeren, Cindy Morgan, Loudell Snow, Gwen Wyatt, and Nancy Ainsworth-Vaughn. That center and some related work at Michigan State was generously funded through the Fetzer Institute of Kalamazoo, and I want at this time to acknowledge the support of Fetzer in helping to develop some of the ideas presented here.

More recently, I have benefited greatly from attending two conferences—one at Harvard University on interdisciplinary approaches to the placebo effect and another sponsored by the Office of Alternative Medicine of the National Institutes of Health on the role of the placebo effect in the scientific study of alternative medicine. I want to thank Anne Harrington, Steven Hyman, Stephen Kosslyn, Dan Moerman, and Wayne Jonas for including me in these conferences, as well as all the attendees who have taught me so much and whose works I have cited.

When it came time actually to write this book, I was aided by Dr. Pamela Peeke, a former medical school classmate now at the NIH, to locate the Gail Ross Literary Agency. Gail Ross and her associate, Howard Yoon, put a great deal of time and effort into the transformation of a writer who had previously addressed academic audiences only through university presses and professional journals into one whose words might resonate with popular audiences. Through their efforts I was next put in touch with Diane Reverand, Matthew Guma, and the rest of the staff of Cliff Street Books at HarperCollins, who all worked hard to be sure that the transformation was complete and that the book fulfilled its potential.

Besides the staff at HarperCollins, I had the privilege of working with two excellent editors, Neill Bogan and Carolyn Fireside. Both grasped quickly and completely the core ideas of the book, and both were very generous in sharing some of their own personal views on health and illness to help develop some passages that remained obscure. Carolyn, in particular, came on board late in the process and did a superb job of final revision under a grueling deadline.

Finally, I must reiterate a portion of the book's dedication and thank the many patients who have taught me so much over the years. Patients, I have come to believe, are extraordinarily forgiving so long as they sense that I am trying. This has given me the courage to go on trying and to find something that seems to work. A wise physician of bygone days supposedly said, "Listen to the patient; he is trying to tell you the diagnosis." To which I would add, "And probably also the treatment."

INTRODUCTION

The Power of the Mind

This book begins and ends with a mystery—a mystery of healing. So it seems appropriate to lead off the introduction with a riddle: *What do the following case studies have in common?*

- Albert consults his physician about a bothersome cold. Because the condition is viral, his doctor knows antibiotics won't help. But Albert—a bit of a hypochondriac—is sure the cold is turning into pneumonia, although it shows no medical signs of doing so, and he pleads for antibiotics. Considering the distress Albert is displaying, his physician makes a choice and writes him a prescription for what he says is a potent antibiotic. In reality, the "antibiotic" is a simple sugar pill—100 percent medically ineffective. Yet once Albert begins taking the "antibiotic," his cold disappears almost overnight.

- Beatrice, who strongly believes in herbal remedies, purchases a much touted new organic food supplement at a health food store. After taking it for several weeks, she feels considerably more energized—despite the lack of any recognized scientific evidence that the supplement can physiologically affect the body.

- Charles develops cancer and undergoes the standard surgery and chemotherapy. As he believes strongly in the healing powers of the mind, he also begins practicing meditation, thinking positive thoughts, and forgiving all the people against whom he harbored grudges. He also stops blaming himself for contracting the disease, realizing it was a bad break but hardly his fault. Not only does he feel better and enjoy life more, he also remains in remission after several years.

- Danielle has just had surgery to remove her gall bladder. Her hospital room is bright and sunny, with a lovely view of a sweeping, tree-lined lawn, and the nurses are especially kind and attentive. Danielle is up and about and feeling great after only ten days—when most gall bladder patients require a recovery period of three to four weeks.

- Eugene, who suffers from mild high blood pressure, volunteers to be a subject for an eight-week experiment of a new drug for hypertension with possibly fewer side effects. Eugene is informed that half the subjects will receive the new drug, while the other half will be given an inert placebo; neither the physicians nor the subjects will know which is which—but, because the people being tested have only mild hypertension, there's little medical risk for the placebo group, especially with a weekly blood pressure check. At the end of the study, when the investigators break the code, Eugene learns he was in the placebo group. Before he was placed on any medication, Eugene's blood pressure was 150/99. During the study, he learns to his amazement, his pressure dropped to 132/88—while taking only an inert placebo.

Just what is it that Albert, Beatrice, Charles, Danielle, and Eugene have in common? At first glance, you'd probably say, "Nothing at all." Some were given various forms of medication by their physician; others did things on their own. Some of them used conventional medicine, while others turned to alternative solutions. Some consciously thought about their conditions; others were influenced by their environment without even being aware of it. So is the answer to our riddle really "nothing at all?"

Not to me. I'd suggest, by contrast, that there is in fact a commonality in all these cases. It's that mysterious phenomenon of the mind working in tandem with the body to enhance healing: the placebo response. What I mean by the phrase is that when a certain set of circumstances are present (what I'll be calling *the meaning model*), ill persons seem to improve greatly in what at first seems an inexplicable way.

Before we discuss the placebo response further, I'd like to tell you a little about myself and how I came to be associated with it. I am a physician, presently Professor of Family Practice and Philosophy at Michigan State University, where I also serve as Director for the Center for Ethics and Humanities in the Life Sciences, while remaining actively involved in the ongoing care of my own patients. I've also written many papers and several books on various aspects of medicine, but have always given special attention to the placebo response. (My book *Placebos and The Philosophy of Medicine* was one of the first full-length works on the subject.)

Indeed, my journey as a practitioner includes an early interest in the placebo response as an intellectually challenging puzzle. For many years I have read as much as I could about this fascinating aspect of medicine and began theorizing to make all that I had read about the placebo response hang together coherently.

While I was doing this reading and theorizing, I was also learning to treat patients. First, my teachers in medical school and in residency showed me how to treat patients; finally I was far enough along to let the patients themselves start to teach me how to treat them. At first, I did not see a lot of carryover between my fancy theories and my actual practice. I tried hard to listen to people and to treat them respectfully, and I thought my relationships with patients were an especially important part of my ability to diagnose them and help them heal. But I believed this because that's what I had been taught, and not because of my study of the placebo response.

As the years went by, I found myself noticing that certain ways of approaching patients seemed to elicit from them both a higher level of satisfaction and also a stronger effort on their part to get better. I was excited to realize, over time, that the approaches that worked were exactly those approaches that best fit with my theories. As I read more recent research into the physician-patient relationship, I kept seeing the same themes I had earlier identified as part of my theoretical construction of the placebo response. I was seeing, finally, the convergence of theory and practice. The theory that seemed intellectually to make the most sense of the placebo response also turned out to guide me directly to the practical approaches that seemed to make patients better. And, in turn, when I thought most carefully about what I saw working in my own practice—or what I read about in medical studies—I found myself further expanding and developing my theories.

In *The Placebo Response*, I'll present what I've learned—which, as I've said, many more physicians every day are also discovering—in ways that will help you achieve and maintain a heightened level of wellness.

I'll explain that the placebo response occurs when we receive certain types of messages or signals from the environment around us. These messages work in some fashion, at some level, to *alter the meaning* of our state of health or illness. Perhaps, for example, the old meaning we attributed to our illness was, "This is scary, and I don't know what's causing it," while the new meaning is "Now I know this is going to get better." Or perhaps the old meaning was, "No one cares what happens to me." Now the meaning becomes, "People around me seem really concerned about my health."

Often what makes these signals especially important for us is that they're tied to *important human relationships.* Perhaps the message that we'll get better comes from a physician or alternative healer whom we have come to know and trust over the years. Or the hope is provided by a support group whose members have suffered through the same sorts of problems that we have.

What does the body do with these messages of meaning? I suggest that the best way to summarize what science has taught us about the placebo response is to visualize *an inner pharmacy*, which we all possess.

Our bodies are capable of producing many substances which can heal a wide variety of illnesses, and make us feel generally healthier and more energized. When the body simply secretes these substances on its own, we have what is often termed "spontaneous healing." Some of the time, our bodies seem slow to react, and a message from outside can serve as a wake-up call to our inner pharmacy. The placebo response can thus be seen as the reaction of our inner pharmacies to that wake-up call—*the message of new meaning.*

It's important to consider just how this process happens and whether there are methods by which we can take control of the process. I've already used the word "mysterious" to describe the placebo response. Keep this in mind as you go through the book. Medical science has learned a lot about the workings of the placebo response; but there has never been a "breakthrough" discovery equivalent to insulin's reversing the effects of diabetes or antibiotics' ability to cure pneumonia. Instead, there have been many smaller clues—some here, some there. It will be our job, as we go through the book, to pick up these clues one by one and organize them into a lucid, scientifically valid view of the phenomenon that makes sense and that can be used by all of us to powerful positive effect.

Now for a brief overview of the book itself. It's divided into two general parts, which we could call "theory" and "practice." Actually, to be more precise, the first part is a mixture of scientific facts and the theories that seem best to explain and organize those facts, or "clues," as we have been calling them. The second part applies those theories to the practical issues of staying healthy and recovering from illness.

In "theory," we'll look at some more examples of the placebo response in action, and define our terms more precisely. We'll study the history of the placebo response in Western medicine, and see how our medical science got to the point where we are now. We'll see what's known about what sorts of persons respond to placebos and under what circumstances. Then we'll take a closer look at the *inner pharmacy* idea and see what that suggests by way of further understanding.

Next, we'll examine two major scientific theories about how placebos work, *expectancy* and *conditioning,* finding that each offers us some additional clues to the placebo response. We'll go on to study a novel model for understanding the placebo response, the *meaning model,* which we've already briefly alluded to—the idea that a positive placebo response is produced when the meaning we assign to the illness experience changes in a positive direction. We'll look at three dimensions of "meaning," each of which will give us further clues for practical healing methods in the second part of the book. Because the flip side of the meaning model is also true—if meaning changes for us in a negative direction, we could get worse—we'll proceed to the *nocebo effect*, or negative placebo response.

Learning about our various biochemical pathways will give us further clues as to how our brains and bodies translate "meaning" into actual changes in our health. These biochemical pathways, in all likelihood, are the "medicines" dispensed by the inner pharmacy. We'll take stock of which clues to the placebo response are still missing, and how new medical research in the next decade may help to fill in those gaps.

Finally, we'll end the theory section by looking at factors which may confuse scientific research by mimicking the placebo response. These factors have led a few experts to suggest that perhaps the placebo response is really a myth. We'll note that, despite these criticisms, the placebo response rests on a firm scientific foundation.

As we turn to "practice," we'll enter a transition zone and address another aspect of the placebo response: its role at the intersection of conventional and alternative medicine. We'll observe how the inner pharmacy can work alongside of and enhance either sort of healing practice.

Then we'll get going with the more practical steps that you can use for healing work. We'll look at the desire to get better, and forgiveness, of others and of ourselves. We'll provide some checklists to help you assess whether these factors are influencing your health in important ways. We'll discuss the use of stories to change the meaning of health and illness events in our lives. We'll look at how social support groups can enhance the work of the inner pharmacy (or, in a few instances, work against it). We'll investigate in detail one element of the meaning model, achieving a sense of mastery or control over the illness, with several specific exercises to make this easier to do. Finally, we'll look at how a relationship with a trusted healer can stimulate your inner pharmacy, discussing both how to choose such a healer, and how to get the most out of each visit when you have found one.

At the book's conclusion, we'll revisit the idea of the placebo response as mystery. There I will suggest that it's critical for us to retain a sense of awe and wonder when we contemplate this intricate connection of mind and body. If we ever start to treat the placebo response as something we can bend to our will with complete predictability (what I call "the quarter-in-the-slot trap" of imagining we will be healed if we just put the right "coin" in the "slot of the vending machine"), then, ironically, the placebo response will stop working for us. If it *is* going to work for us, it will be partly to the extent that we continue to view it as mysterious.

Even if we cannot absolutely control or guarantee the placebo response, the possibility remains that *we can harness it* to heal faster, stay healthier, and generally function better. And that idea is what I want to leave with you. Along with the concept of the inner pharmacy, it's the most important new concept this book contains. You see, previous writing about the placebo response has treated it as something done *to* you, over which you have little if any control. I'm proposing that, if we line up the scientific clues in the right order, we'll master a variety of means by which we can employ the placebo response and the inner pharmacy to benefit ourselves.

So let's begin our investigation into one of the mind-body's greatest —and most fascinating—mysteries and see what medical puzzles we can solve along the way.

ONE

What Is the Placebo Response?

"One of the most successful physicians I have ever known, has assured me that he used more of bread pills, drops of coloured water, and powders of hickory ashes, than of all other medicines put together."

—THOMAS JEFFERSON (1807)

Medicine usually describes a phenomenon before defining it formally, and that has been the case with the *placebo response;* the quotation above, for example, demonstrates that nearly two hundred years ago there was an awareness of the mind's powerful influence over the body's illness and healing. In the course of this book, you'll be reading many stories that provide new clues to various aspects of the mysterious phenomenon we call the placebo response: aspects such as *expectancy*, *conditioning*, and *meaning*.

Briefly, *expectancy* refers to changes in bodily health which occur because we anticipate they will happen. *Conditioning* refers to the way repeated past experiences create a pattern of bodily change which may be replicated in the present. And *meaning*, which I mentioned in the introduction, refers to the way we interpret and try to make sense of the events that befall us. (In chapter 7, we'll look at some of the elements that comprise meaning, as well as the connection between the meaning of events and the stories we tell about them.) The case studies that follow dramatically illustrate these three aspects of the placebo response.

Mr. Wright, Krebiozen, and the Newspaper Headlines

One of the most often-repeated stories about the placebo response is a case reported by a colleague to Dr. Bruno Klopfer and published by Klopfer in 1957. As a single incident, it must be interpreted with skepticism; but the facts are so intriguing, it's difficult to discount. Klopfer's colleague was the personal physician of a patient, known as "Mr. Wright," who was suffering from cancer of the lymph system and had developed large tumors throughout his body that could easily be felt by his doctors.

At the time, a group of physicians were studying a new chemical formula called krebiozen, which was being widely touted by the media as a miracle cure for cancer—although the medical establishment was less convinced. Wright's cancer was so far advanced that the physicians initially considered excluding him from the research study, but finally gave him the drug as a compassionate exception—not because they expected any response. What happened next truly seemed like a miracle. Mr. Wright gained weight, looked and felt better, and his tumors shrank so drastically, they could hardly be detected.

Wright's improvement continued until local newspapers began reporting krebiozen was not the great advance it had first been thought. After reading the negative coverage, Mr. Wright became discouraged, immediately began to lose weight, and his tumors grew once more.

Assuming that the power of suggestion had been largely responsible for Mr. Wright's response to the medication, the physicians decided to tell him that the first batches of krebiozen sent to their clinic had not been at full potency. The lab had corrected the problem, they assured him, and the new, stronger batch of the drug would soon be on its way. They continued to encourage Mr. Wright's hopes, finally announcing that the big day was here—the new batch of the drug had arrived. They then proceeded to give Mr. Wright injections just as before—*using sterile water.*

Being treated only with sterile water, Mr. Wright showed the same dramatic improvements that had occurred with the krebiozen. His remission lasted until, for a second time, the newspapers undermined the physicians—stating unequivocally that "AMA reports that krebiozen is worthless against cancer." Mr. Wright once again began to sink, his tumors grew massive, and shortly thereafter, he died.

Mr. Wright's story illustrates the importance of *expectancy* in determining whether or not a placebo response will occur. The next case demonstrates *conditioning*, by showing that the placebo response may depend not only on what we expect to happen in the future, but also what *has happened* to us in the past.

Ruth's Rose Perfume

Working with Dr. Karen Olness in Cleveland, Robert Ader of the University of Rochester assisted in treating a young teenager named "Ruth," who had developed a severe case of systemic lupus erythematosis when she was eleven. Two years later, she was suffering from kidney damage, high blood pressure, and bleeding as a result of this severe autoimmune disease. Her physicians decided that she required immediate treatment with the powerful drug cyclophosphamide to shut off her overactive immune system.

Ruth's mother, a psychologist, knew that Ader (whom we'll read more about in chapter 6) had done experiments with cyclophosphamide on rats. In these experiments, the rats had received a harmless but distinctive substance along with the cyclophosphamide. Later, when they got the harmless substance alone, their bodies reacted as if they had received another dose of the cyclophosphamide. Ruth's mother wondered if a similar method could be used to reduce the amount of cyclophosphamide her daughter would be receiving—possibly sparing her the medicine's toxic side effects. The physicians agreed to this trial, eventually pairing the cyclophosphamide treatment with two other distinctive substances: cod liver oil and a strong rose perfume.

For three months Ruth received full-dose treatments with cyclophosphamide; she was also given cod liver oil and allowed to smell the perfume during each monthly treatment. At later monthly treatments, she continued to receive the cod liver oil and the perfume, but the cyclophosphamide was administered in only one out of three sessions. Therefore, in the course of a year, Ruth received half the total dose of cyclophosphamide she would normally have gotten. Despite this she had an excellent response, and her lupus went into a remission.

Both expectancy and conditioning, as I've mentioned, relate to another key aspect of the placebo response: *meaning.* What does illness and the process of healing *mean* to the person who is sick? Often this meaning is worked out or expressed through communication within the *relationship* with a doctor or other healer, as the following anecdote demonstrates.

The Importance of Listening

In the mid-80s, a group of family physicians in Canada, led by Dr. Martin Bass, performed a fascinating study of a large group of patients coming to family doctors with a wide array of common symptoms. The investigators basically asked one question: What best predicts whether this patient will say that she is better if we come back one month later and ask her about her illness?

Somewhat to the embarrassment of the medical establishment, their detailed review of the medical charts showed a lot of things that did *not* predict whether the patient would get better. The thoroughness of the medical history and physical exam, whether the physician did any lab tests or X rays, and which medications were prescribed had nothing to do with the outcome after one month. In fact, almost everything physicians are taught in medical school and residency turned out to make no difference for this group of patients.

However, Bass and his colleagues were able to identify the one factor that best predicted whether the patient would report feeling better after one month: whether the patient stated that the physician had carefully listened to his description of his condition at the first office visit.

Bass and colleagues also identified a large group of patients who came in with the new onset of headache, and followed those patients for an entire year. After one year, they found that what best predicted an improvement in the headaches was the patients' report that at the very first visit, they had a chance to discuss their problem fully and felt the physician was able to appreciate what it meant to them. (And if you think the finding might be a fluke, consider that Barbara Starfield of Johns Hopkins University did a similar study of public health clinic patients in Baltimore and reached exactly the same conclusion.)

But I must note here that meaning can go two ways, one of them downhill.

The Nocebo Response: Flip Side of the Coin

What happens when a sick person like Mr. Wright attaches a negative rather than a positive meaning to the attempt at treatment? This negative mind-set can be so strong, it's been given its own name: the *nocebo response.* We'll be discussing the nocebo effect in greater detail later on; meanwhile, here's another example of the tremendous power of negativity.

A Woman Who Died of Abbreviation

Of the various case reports which support the idea of the nocebo response, one of the more compelling was recorded by a renowned cardiologist, Dr. Bernard Lown.

Early in his career, Dr. Lown was working under a very distinguished senior cardiologist, who in turn was taking care of a woman, Mrs. S., with a non-life-threatening heart-valve condition called tricuspid stenosis. She also suffered from a mild degree of congestive heart failure, which was successfully controlled with medication. At the time of the precipitating event, Mrs. S. was in the hospital to have some tests done, and was in her usual stable condition.

One day, the senior cardiologist came into her room, accompanied by a bevy of residents, interns, and medical students. As was customary in those days (and still is, far too often, in teaching hospitals today), the group talked among themselves—treating the patient as if she were an object, paying no direct attention to her, and excluding her from their conversation. Before the whole mob turned on their heels and filed out of the room, the senior physician announced, "This woman has TS"—employing an abbreviation cardiologists commonly use for "tricuspid stenosis."

Dr. Lown came back to see Mrs. S. shortly thereafter and was stunned to find her anxious, frightened, and breathing very rapidly. Her lungs, which had been perfectly clear a couple of hours before, now displayed the moist crackling noises in the lower portions which portended a worsening of the congestive heart failure. When Lown asked Mrs. S. what was the matter, she replied, "That doctor said that I was going to die for sure."

Lown could not believe what he was hearing, and protested that his senior couldn't possibly have made such a statement. "I heard him," Mrs. S. replied firmly. "He said I had TS. I know that means 'terminal situation.' You doctors never tell us the truth straight out. You always try to hide it to soften the blow. But I know what he meant."

Even Lown's insistence that by "TS" his senior had meant "tricuspid stenosis," not "terminal situation," had no effect on Mrs. S. She quietly reiterated that she knew perfectly well what was going on, and that Dr. Lown was simply trying to shield her from the awful truth. After the incident, she continued to slide into worse and worse heart failure, despite the total lack of objective evidence that anything fundamental had changed in her underlying heart condition. She passed away later that same day.

Such is the power of negative meaning. Still, my own interest in the placebo response is chiefly positive, centered in its ability to heal. So I ask: Could harboring hope, faith, or expectation be genuinely potent factors in the healing process? I believe they are. In fact, I see them as the heart and soul of the placebo response.

I'll continue using "placebo response" rather broadly to include many diverse healing events reported by medical scientists and observers over centuries. Since we've established that the placebo response embraces many different facets—as we saw in the cases of Albert, Beatrice, Charles, Danielle, and Eugene in the introduction—let's explore in more detail just what it is.

Defining *Placebo* and *Placebo Response*

The placebo response seems to be the body's reaction to some healing signal in the environment, which acts through the mind. What might a "healing signal" be? Consider the general concept of a *symbol.* The concept has a number of features that seem to make it very useful for explaining the sort of signal we are talking about.

- Many different things in the environment can serve as symbols: a word, a picture, a gesture, to name but a few.

- For something to serve as a symbol, the receiving person has to be in a certain state of mind, and to have had a certain history. A word is not a symbol unless we know its language. A flag, for instance, is not a symbol unless we recognize it as pertaining to a nation with which we have some ties of emotion or loyalty; otherwise it is merely a colored piece of cloth.

- We usually call something a symbol when it stands for or invokes something much more powerful or vast than the thing itself. If someone didn't understand the sense in which a flag is the patriotic symbol of a nation, she would never comprehend why raising aloft that piece of colored cloth sent masses of soldiers rushing forward to risk death on the battlefield. (If the traditional placebo seems to be "inert" all by itself, and yet somehow has the capacity to unleash very powerful responses, we can understand this by viewing the placebo *as a symbol.*)

- A symbol can affect us either consciously or unconsciously. Imagine that I hear the theme music from a horror movie that I watched as a small child. I might easily find myself sweating and my heart racing—and this could happen even if I have no conscious memory of seeing the film.

- Though responses to symbols can be unconscious, we generally assume that a fairly complex mind is required to understand and respond to symbols, and especially to create symbols. That is, we would not expect to see symbols having any impact on lower animals with very primitive mental abilities. We'd expect symbols to be potent only in humans or in animals sufficiently like us in mental capacity.

- The same thing can function as a symbol and as something else. For instance, consider a slap on the face, in the old days of dueling. We might ask a person who had been slapped why he felt wounded, and there would be two answers. The slap itself, shorn of any symbolic meaning, is a physical reason to feel localized pain. But the slap is also a symbol for domination and humiliation, which could be emotionally very painful. Thus, something can function as a symbol without disqualifying it from having a bodily effect by another route.

- Symbols can be especially powerful when they serve to remind us of important human relationships. In chapter 6, when we discuss conditioning theory in detail, we'll look at the possibility that the earliest example of conditioning in most of our lives may be when our mothers fed us substances to make us healthy (like chicken soup), or kissed a boo-boo, or put a Band-Aid on it. The Band-Aid may have become for us as children a very powerful symbol of healing—but would it have been anywhere near as powerful without its ability to remind us of the extremely important relationship with Mother? In this way, symbols might help explain why the most powerful placebo responses are in one way or another often embedded in important human relationships.

Therefore, something has *symbolic significance* for us when it makes us think or feel differently—because we interpret the symbol as representing something bigger than, or beyond, its mere physical characteristics. So I can now expand my definition of *placebo response* to:

> ***A change in the body (or the body-mind unit) that occurs as the result of the symbolic significance which one attributes to an event or object in the healing environment.***

Let's review several features of this definition.

- Notice that the definition refers to a *change*. As we've seen, this could be positive or negative; so the placebo response can make one worse as well as better.

- The stipulation "in the healing environment" is intended to draw a boundary around the notion of placebo response. We are assuming that the placebo response is the result of some sort of mind-body process. Do we want to call every possible way the mind could influence the body a placebo response? For instance, workers in a company go to a motivational seminar and as a result work harder, so that the company turns a hefty profit. Is that a placebo response? Not according to my definition.

  I propose that the placebo response, despite the fact that it is a relatively wide concept, should be restricted to certain sorts of mind-body interactions: those that occur within a healing context (which, as we will see below, may include self-care).

- The placebo response is not restricted to symbols or signals which have no other possible impact on the body. A pill, injection, or surgical procedure, for instance, could easily have *both* a direct effect on the body by means understood by the usual biomedical theories, and also a symbolic impact which gives rise to a placebo response.

- The definition does not regard physical and mental treatments as being in fundamentally different categories. We think that a sugar pill, if it causes bodily change, can do so only through a symbolic effect, because it lacks the power to work in any other way.

  On the other hand, if we take cimetidine (Tagamet) for an ulcer, it has the potential to work in at least two ways: it can reduce stomach acid secretion by turning off specific chemical processes in certain stomach cells; and it can exert a placebo effect like any other pill or capsule. Similarly, if we undergo psychotherapy and our anxiety or depression gets better, it could be because the psychotherapy works on specific psychological processes directly; it doesn't have to stand for anything else. But the psychotherapy could also function as a placebo, to the extent, for instance, that the patient expects to get better with psychotherapy and views it as powerful treatment, or feels especially cared for and supported by the therapist. The same would be true of any alternative healing practice.

- This definition excludes from the placebo response the common process which is usually referred to as "spontaneous healing" or the natural history of the disease process, which, we assume, might well occur without any events of special symbolic significance. Few illnesses are fatal, even if the sufferer never sees a physician—and even if the sufferer never takes as much as one aspirin tablet or herbal remedy. The normal course of most illnesses is to get better even without any healing intervention, whether from a healer or from oneself. I do not include these improvements in the body's placebo responses. (We'll see in chapter 10 a list of other factors that could mimic the placebo response.)

The Placebo Response and Its Myths

How one ought to define "placebo response" has been extremely controversial. (Indeed, some experts have suggested that one *cannot* define it in any logically coherent way.) Now that I have told you how I think the term should be defined, and why that definition makes the most sense, I want to turn briefly to some definitional approaches which seem to me to be unsatisfactory. I mention them for two reasons. First, dispensing with the myths about the placebo response helps us understand it more clearly. Second, if you further research the subject, you're likely to run into these terms, and so it pays to be familiar with their shortcomings.

Inert treatment. Placebo is often defined as a medical substance or treatment which is inactive or inert. If we assume that a placebo is something like a sugar pill or a syringe full of sterile water, that description seems to work. The sciences of biochemistry and pharmacology teach us that those substances, in those amounts, are indeed inert in terms of their ability to affect the body in a direct, purely chemical way. But notice how misleading this word "inert" is, even if we restrict ourselves to sugar pills and water injections, which is a very limited subset of all the things that interest us.

First, if placebos were really inert, in the sense of doing absolutely nothing to change the body of the sick person, I wouldn't have written this book and you wouldn't be reading it. The problem of defining "placebo" arises precisely because the placebo *does* produce changes, no matter how enigmatic they may seem.

Second, if placebos do change the body, it seems hard to imagine how they could do so *without* involving chemical pathways of one sort or another. After all, everything else that happens in the body—including thinking and feeling—is associated with measurable physical and chemical changes. To say that placebos affect the body's health, but that they somehow do it without altering the body's chemistry, is much more mysterious (and less scientific) than to postulate that the placebo operates on the body by some chemical routes. (In chapter 9, I'll discuss which ones these might be.)

Nonspecific responses. Because "inert" is misleading, some placebo scientists have chosen the term "nonspecific effects." This expression has even appeared as the title of one book about placebos. Some scientists view "nonspecific response" as virtually synonymous with "placebo response"; others would say that the placebo response is just one type of nonspecific response.

Just what is meant by "nonspecific effect"? Since often no formal definition is given, let's look at the contrasting term, "specific effect." *A specific effect* is presumably a change in the body that occurs as a direct causal outcome of some medical action; and we possess a well-grounded theory in medical science to explain exactly why that action should affect the body in a certain way. Resolution of bacterial pneumonia as a result of injecting antibiotics; lowering of a diabetic's blood sugar when insulin is administered; the shrinkage of a tumor after radiation treatments—all would count as "specific effects." An effect, then, might be "nonspecific" either because the causal link between the medical action and the effect is uncertain, or because our existing theories do not establish precisely why it should occur at all.

"Nonspecific," then, looks better to the scientific mind because it is open-ended: It refuses to assume that we know what causes placebo responses if we really don't. Also, some see the very term "placebo" as confusing, precisely because it carries so much baggage with it; thus, removing "placebo" from the definition makes the whole idea cleaner. (We'll discuss in chapters 2 and 3 why "placebo" has come to have a negative connotation for many experts.)

But "nonspecific" won't work as well as its advocates think. Until you can list exactly what the other nonspecific responses are, and then show how the placebo response resembles them, you have really not said anything interesting.

I have an even more serious objection to "nonspecific response." In the sense that most of us would think of using the term, the placebo response *is not* nonspecific. Imagine, for instance, that physicians give sugar pills to two groups of patients. One group is suffering from pain and the other is suffering from asthma. The first group is told that the sugar pills are analgesics; the second is told that the pills are bronchodilators to help them breathe more easily.

Based on what we know about such placebo experiments, we can say with confidence that at least some of the first group of patients are likely to report that they have less pain; and some of the second group are likely to report that they can breathe more easily and have less wheezing. What we would *not* expect is for some of the second group to report that the asthma is just as bad, but they have less pain; or for some of the first group to say that they can breathe more easily even though their pain is no better. So, based on all the available evidence from a large number of studies, the placebo response appears to be quite specific for the disease or symptom being treated and for the sort of treatment the patient expects to receive. (This is precisely why, as we will see in chapter 5, *expectancy* is such an important aspect of understanding the placebo response.) If this is so, then defining the placebo response as some sort of "nonspecific response" is inaccurate as well as uninformative.

The Independence of Placebo Response from Placebo

You'll notice that so far, we have been defining *placebo response,* but we have said almost nothing about defining *placebo.* A *placebo,* in common medical parlance, is a dummy pill or form of medical treatment that apparently contains no substance that is active in fighting against whatever disease the patient has. A commonly used placebo pill today contains 100 milligrams of lactose, or milk sugar, and Western science denies that this could possibly alter the body's internal chemistry enough to affect the course of any disease.

The definition I proposed earlier, by introducing the concept of symbolic significance, allows me to define placebo *response* as if it were independent from the notion of placebo. This will turn out to be very important when we get to practical applications.

Historically, medicine first discovered the effect of symbolic significance on health by seeing improvement in patients who were given bread pills, sugar pills, or other dummy medicines that could exert *only* a symbolic power. Today, we need not be limited by that history. We

Colorado Mountain College
Alpine Campus Library
1330 Bob Adams Drive
Steamboat Springs, CO 80487

must realize that virtually every time a healer administers a treatment to a person with an illness, or every time an individual treats herself for an illness with some healing substance or process, the individual receives messages from the environment which, if they possess the correct symbolic significance, may trigger a placebo response. Of all the placebo responses occurring presently, only a tiny percentage arise as the result of giving a treatment which could accurately be termed a placebo.

In order to finish up properly, we should define precisely what a placebo is, even if it is at this time relegated to the back bench as a way to elicit a placebo response:

> ***In medical research, a placebo is an intervention designed to mimic the modality or process being studied, but without any of its nonsymbolic healing properties, so as to serve as a control in a double-blind trial (in which the control group gets a dummy treatment, and neither the subjects nor the investigators know which group gets the active treatment and which gets the dummy).***
>
> ***In therapeutic healing, a placebo is a treatment modality or process administered with the belief that it possesses the ability to affect the body only by virtue of its symbolic significance.***

By defining our terms in such a way that the placebo response does not depend in any way on administering placebos, we have cleared the path for completely ethical, nondeceptive communications between the healer and the patient. If communicating with the patient in a certain way promotes better healing, there is no reason whatever why the practitioner cannot say this right up front—and indeed there is no reason why the practitioner cannot teach some of these aspects of communication to the patient.

This understanding will lead directly to the major themes to be discussed in the remainder of the book. You'll see how the idea of the inner pharmacy serves as a central image to capture the essence of the placebo response. You'll study the evidence that the pharmacy is affected by what we expect to happen in the future (expectancy), as well as by the patterns of things that have happened to us repeatedly in the past (conditioning). You'll comprehend why that pharmacy should be especially influenced by the meaning we attach to events in our lives, and to how those events are embedded within important human relationships. And finally you'll learn how all that leads to a program for taking charge of your own inner pharmacies to use its power for your own healing.

As I have said, the way we defined our terms in this chapter means that we need not be limited by the history of deceptive use of placebos. It is just that history which I will explore in the next chapter.

TWO

The Placebo Response: A Historical Perspective

"Since almost all medications until recently were placebos, the history of medical treatment can be characterized largely as the history of the placebo effect."

—Arthur K. Shapiro, 1968

It's useful to gain a quick historical overview of the placebo response by studying what physicians and other experts were doing and saying about it during earlier centuries. Here's a provocative account from 1580.

The Rich Merchant's Magic Enema

Michel de Montaigne, the great French essayist, wrote about the power of the imagination to influence the body's functioning four hundred years ago. In one essay, he recounted a story which had been told to him by an apothecary (we would call him a pharmacist).

There lived in Toulouse a rich merchant, who was so greatly troubled with bladder stones that he had become an invalid. This merchant had enormous faith in enemas (or clysters, as they were then called), and over the years persuaded his physicians to prescribe him a vast quantity and variety—depending on the precise symptoms he was feeling at any given time.

On one occasion, when he called for a particular kind of clyster, the apothecary and his assistants went through the customary ritual: arranging him in the proper position in bed, carefully checking the temperature of the admixture, up to and including inserting the syringe into the merchant's rectum. The apothecary and his assistants then departed, but the next morning called on the merchant to inquire about the results of the previous day's procedure. He exclaimed that things had worked wonderfully, just as always. But what the merchant didn't know is that on this occasion, the apothecary had only *pretended* to inject his patient with the solution.

What the apothecary did is clear. Why he did it is not—Montaigne's essay provides no clues as to the motive. I suspect it was a private joke played by the apothecary on an overly demanding patient.

Let's next turn our attention to the two divergent schools of thought which have dominated medicine down through the centuries.

Spontaneous Healing vs. Powers of the Imagination: The Historical Debate

The placebo response has always been a part of medicine and healing. For us to learn as much as we can from that history, we need to ask whether physicians and healers of those earlier times ever used placebos or the placebo effect; and if so, how they imagined these processes worked. Let's start by investigating medical treatments that work even when they don't adhere to the prevailing healing theory of the day.

Each period in medical history has had its favorite treatments and cures. Often there was little if any evidence—of the sort we'd consider valid today—that these treatments made any real difference. Still, medicine has always tried to be scientific in some sense. That means constructing a theory of how various treatments affected the body to eliminate or reduce the effects of disease and restore health. Such ancient treatments as crocodile dung or powdered mummy may seem ridiculous to us today, but to the physicians who used them, there was logic to why they were used and how they were expected to function.

What did physicians do, then, when a treatment seemed to heal the patient—but its effect couldn't be explained by the predominant theory of the day? Throughout the history of medicine, there been have two major answers provided by physicians, which I discussed in chapter 1: the healing power of hope, faith, and the imagination (what I am calling the placebo response); and the inherent healing power of the body itself (spontaneous healing).

One of the first authorities to write about the healing powers of the imagination was not a physician at all, but the Greek philosopher Plato, who leaned toward the belief that words could have healing powers and that the spoken word's influence on an ill patient's mind might lead to a cure. Plato was even willing to consider that such words might literally be a lie: for example, a physician expressing confidence that a seriously ill patient will recover or that the disease is not as grave as the man imagines. By accepting the legitimacy of the lie in medical circumstances, Plato exempted physicians from the society's normal bias against lying because he believed the medical lie might be a critical part of the healing practice:

> ***"Again, a high value must be set upon truthfulness. If we were right in saying the gods have no use for falsehood and that it is useful to mankind only in the way of a medicine, obviously a medicine should be handled by no one but a physician."***

Plato's opinions about persuasion by the physician over the patient could be contrasted with those of a famous Greek authority on the subject: Hippocrates, "the father of modern medicine" (although his writings were probably not the work of one man, but of a school of associates and disciples). Hippocrates doesn't seem to accept the notion that persuasion or the idea of the "word" could promote healing by itself. Rather, he believes that if the physician persuades the patient, he will dutifully take his medicine and follow any advice given by the physician; thus, close adherence to the proper treatment acts as the healing agent. Although Plato and Hippocrates have apparently diverging views, the philosopher, in *The Laws*, seems to agree with the physician:

> ***"The free physician—the one who does not attend to slaves—shares his impressions with the patients and the latter's friends; while he informs himself about the patient at the same time (insofar as possible), he instructs him and prescribes nothing without persuading him beforehand. Thus, with the aid of persuasion, he soothes and continually disposes him so as to lead him little by little to health."***

The next great Greek physician, Galen, propounded a theory which would dominate Western medicine for the subsequent 1800 years. Galen's theory, humoral medicine, shares important commonalities with traditional Chinese and Hindu ayurvedic medicines. These disciplines all emphasize the presence in the body of a small number of elements. The body is healthy when the elements are balanced and in harmony; disease occurs when there is an elemental imbalance. So medicine's role is to restore balance—either by helping to decrease an element which is excessive or by strengthening an element which is deficient. Even today, the concept of harmony and balance is key to many alternative medical systems.

Humoral medicine, as taught by Galen, considered there to be four types of elements or bodily fluids called humors—blood, phlegm, black bile, and yellow bile—and was quite "holistic" from a mind-body perspective. That is, mental influences were thought to be just as capable as any physical cause of affecting the balance of the humors, for good or ill. Words such as "sanguine," "melancholy," and "phlegmatic" refer today to personality types or psychological traits, but they originally meant an excess of one of the four humors (blood, black bile, yellow bile, and phlegm, respectively).

Because of the holism of the humoral theory, it was quite easy for physicians during its 1800 year reign to credit the emotions or the imagination with producing cures or causing disease or deformity. Some physicians were even-handed on this issue, admitting that the mind could be at least partially responsible for any cure. Read Dr. Jerome Gaub, writing in 1763:

> ***"[H]ope . . . buoys up a mind enfeebled by an obstinate tedious ailment and want of help. The arousal of the bodily organs is sometimes such that the vital principles cast off their torpidity, the tone of the nervous system is restored, the movements of the humors are accelerated, and nature then attacks and overcomes with her powers a disease that prolonged treatment had opposed in vain."***

Others insisted that imagination was responsible for the cures done by quacks or charlatans (or with whomever they disagreed), while their own cures were due to nothing but great skill and learning. In his *Anatomy of Melancholy* (1628), Robert Burton quoted several famous authorities on the subject from earlier periods:

> ***"There is no virtue in such charms or cures (used by quacks), but a strong conceit and opinion alone, as Pomponatius holds, 'which forceth a motion of the humors, spirits, and blood, which takes away the cause of the malady from the parts affected.' . . . 'Tis opinion alone (saith Cardan) that makes or mars physicians, and he doth the best cures, according to Hippocrates, in whom most trust.'"***

When, in this long period of medical history, did physicians first begin to administer treatments they knew to be "dummies," just so they could produce a cure due solely to the imagination? I doubt anybody knows, but the case of "The Rich Merchant's Magic Enema," reported, you'll recall, in 1580, is the earliest reference to a deliberate dummy treatment I've been able to find.

Let's turn now to the derivation and evolution of the placebo.

The Placebo's Fall from Grace

The word "placebo" itself means "I shall please" in Latin and first appeared in English usage in the early Middle Ages, referring to vespers sung for the dead. By the time of the poet Chaucer, in the fourteenth century, "placebo" had acquired the negative connotation which has dogged it ever since. Then it referred to a flatterer or yes-man, who would always tell you what you wanted to hear, never what he really thought to be true.

Centuries would pass before "placebo" acquired medical associations. It was not until 1785 that it entered the scientific lexicon as a type of medicine—and not until 1811 would a definition appear that even remotely resembles our sense of the word today. Although Thomas Jefferson was fully aware in 1807 that in using "bread pills, drops of coloured water, and powders of hickory ashes," his physician friend was trying to influence the mind and not the body of the patient, it probably wouldn't have occurred to him to use the word "placebo" for these substances.

It was also around the time of the American Revolution that we first see the use of a control group in a medical experiment. Credit for the invention of the "blind" control may belong to another one of our founding fathers, Benjamin Franklin.

Dr. Franklin and Mr. Mesmer

One of the hottest fads in the Paris of 1784 was "animal magnetism" (or "mesmerism"), developed by Franz Anton Mesmer. Today we know the process as "hypnotism," but Mesmer claimed that mesmerism's power derived from a newly discovered natural bodily fluid. His special techniques for putting subjects in a trance and transmitting suggestions, he insisted, depended on his ability to manipulate this fluid in the subject, from a distance.

When the King of France appointed a scientific commission to inquire into the validity of Mesmer's theory, Franklin, then the American minister to France, was asked to be a member. The commission first decided on a focal issue: Was animal magnetism truly a natural, physical force, or were its effects owed purely to the mesmerist's prowess at stimulating the subject's imagination? Franklin and his associates determined this by imposing blind conditions and found that in each case they could eliminate the effects of the animal magnetism.

For instance, women who had been mesmerized could say very accurately where in their bodies they felt the magnetic fluid, as long as they could see the mesmerist. As soon as they were blindfolded, their answers became totally random. In another set of experiments, the women were told that the mesmerist was behind a curtain in an adjoining room, which might have been true or false. The commission observed that the subjects' ability to be mesmerized depended on their *thinking he was there*—and not on whether he was actually present.

After several sets of these experiments Franklin and his fellow commissioners concluded that it was the imagination of the subjects, and not any fluid, that could best account for the effects of mesmerism.

The Tractor Test

A related experimental technique was used in England in 1799 to expose what traditional physicians regarded as yet another quack remedy. An American doctor, Elisha Perkins, had introduced metal "tractors," small rods resembling a drawing compass which were supposed to act on the body's electrical fields. People with paralyzed limbs and other severe disorders claimed to be dramatically healed after the use of the tractors.

When the "tractors" were imported into England, Dr. John Haygarth and his colleagues—aware of Franklin's methods—developed phony wooden tractors, painted to look like metal. Using these dummies, they succeeded in "curing" fifteen British patients.

Around 1834, the French doctor Armand Trousseau appears to have been the first to use what we would today call a *placebo control,* in studies designed to test (and to reject) the claims of the rising homeopathic school of medicine. Trousseau and his students realized that to control adequately for the homeopathic remedies, another similar group of patients needed to receive a dummy which appeared identical. They decided on bread pills.

At that time, no one even thought of revealing to the experimental subjects what was being done—as is now required in all ethical experiments. Trousseau's group, biased from the start, concluded that homeopathy was medically useless, and that its patients' health improved because of the natural history of their illnesses.

By 1811, just as we start to see the word "placebo" actually used in medicine, we also witness some tension about what the placebo is supposed to accomplish. Many nineteenth-century physicians assumed that, if a cure was not caused by a specific remedy, it must be caused by the body's inherent healing powers—not necessarily the imagination. In 1898, Dr. Elmer Lee wrote:

> ***"The principal influence or relation [of drugs] to the cure of bodily disease lies in the fact that drugs supply material on which to rest the mind while other agencies are at work eliminating the disease from the system, and so the drug is frequently given the credit."***

Dr. Flint's Placeboic Remedy

The American physician Austin Flint, for example, set out to prove that most of the treatments then used for rheumatic fever were useless, and that patients improved equally if left totally on their own. But Flint's patients in New York's Bellevue Hospital didn't want simply to be observed; they demanded treatment. Flint obliged by giving them a special medicine he called "the placeboic remedy"—actually a highly diluted tincture of a bitter-tasting tropical bark called quassia, which was totally inactive for the disease. He even used the term "placeboic remedy" with the subjects, concluding correctly that most of them had never heard of placebo. To the subjects, "placeboic remedy" was simply the name of the new medicine.

As he expected, Flint found that patients treated with the "placeboic remedy" got better at approximately the same rate as patients treated with the then-popular remedies for rheumatic fever. Flint stopped there, never considering the possibility that he was influencing the patients' minds or imaginations and thereby effecting faster cures. He simply assumed that by giving the tincture of quassia, he was observing the natural history of the disease, precisely as if he and Bellevue Hospital didn't exist.

Now let's explore the other prevailing historical theory: the mind's ability to effect a cure.

The Healing Imagination

Alongside the belief in the body's inherent healing powers, belief in the power of the imagination persisted. As evidence accumulated during the nineteenth century, it became more difficult to claim that the effect seen when placebos were given was the result only of the inherent healing powers of the body. When Dr. Horatio C. Wood reported the following case in 1891, he assumed that the patient's imagination accounted for the results:

> ***"Some time ago I gave a patient, with very minute and emphatic instructions as to the method of use, a prescription for pills of bread. Several months after she came back to me and said, 'Doctor, why did you not give me that prescription sooner? It is the only thing that has reached my case, and I have had that prescription filled at the apothecary's for a number of my friends with extraordinary results.'"***

Uncertainty over how to explain the success of the placebo—whether by the body's inherent healing powers or by the imagination—did not cause physicians to be leery of using placebos deliberately in practice. Charles Rosenberg, a prominent medical historian, writes:

> ***"No mid–19th century physician doubted the efficacy of placebos (as little as he doubted that the effectiveness of a drug could depend on his own manner and attitude) . . . "***

Indeed, it appears (though exact statistics are unavailable) that a great quantity of placebos were deliberately dispensed by physicians in the nineteenth and early twentieth century. Richard Cabot, a prominent Harvard physician, wrote in 1903:

> ***"Now I was brought up, as I suppose every physician is, to use placebos, bread pills, water subcutaneously, and other devices for acting on a patient's symptoms through his mind. How frequently such methods are used varies a great deal I suppose with individual practitioners, but I doubt if there is a physician in this room who has not used them and used them pretty often."***

And even as late as 1953, the editor of the *British Medical Journal* would say:

> ***"[At a recent meeting of the General Practice Section of the Royal Society of Medicine in England, the discussion suggested that general practitioners may prescribe placebos for patients at about 40 percent of visits.] In 1949, 188 million prescriptions were dispensed in England. If 40 percent of these prescriptions were for a placebo [and using 4 ounces of a typical placebo mixture as the basis for calculation], the annual cost of dispensing placebos would amount to 5–3/4 million pounds."***

Widely prescribed or not, placebos have always been at the center of a storm of controversy, on ethical grounds.

Medical Ethics and the Placebo Response

Since many nineteenth- and early twentieth-century physicians compounded their own medicines, they could hand the patient the bottle of pills without anyone else knowing what was in them (covering them up with fancy Latin names), making it easy to prescribe placebos deceptively. As we have seen, the prevailing ethical standards of those days permitted physicians lying to their patients, as long as the goal was healing, not making money.

Physicians were also prompted to prescribe placebos because they came increasingly to recognize that few available medicines were genuinely effective in healing. This led Dr. John Snow, a pioneer scientific investigator in anesthesiology and epidemiology, to predict confidently in 1855 that placebo use would disappear as medicine became more scientific and as the effects of treatment became more predictable:

> ***"Some branches of medical science have already attained a great amount of certainty; surgeons, for instance, are in agreement about the proper treatment of fractures and dislocations. . . . [When] the nature and treatment of [all] diseases becomes equally well known, it will be impossible that intelligent persons should submit to being treated with globules of sugar of milk, having the name of medicine attached to them, and nothing else."***

As the twentieth century proceeded, deliberate use of placebos in medical practice declined, as physicians now had considerably more faith that they could prescribe effective medication for their patients' problems. In addition, patients started to ask more questions and to demand more information. Lawyers began suing physicians for failing to obtain a patient's informed consent to treatment. Ethical standards in medicine were changing dramatically, and deceiving patients no longer seemed prudent. Dr. Norman Shure, writing in 1965, had decidedly mixed feelings about the concept of *placebo surgery* (about which I'll explain more later):

> ***"I knew a surgeon years ago who thought nothing of performing an oblique lower right quadrant incision, then suturing without entering the abdominal cavity in patients who had emotional problems manifested by pain in the abdomen. His results were excellent and as one might expect his operative mortality and morbidity were exceptionally low. . . . Certainly this is not common and I doubt whether anyone else would have done such pro-***

cedures. However I am certain that thousands of appendectomies and hysterectomies are done yearly as placebos."

Even today, one occasionally finds placebos used in American hospitals or clinics. In many of these instances, the use is justified by a common myth: that the placebo is a kind of aid in medical diagnosis. Many physicians still believe (contrary to the evidence we will be reviewing in later chapters) that the *only time* a placebo can relieve pain is when the pain is purely "imaginary." When a patient is suspected, then, to have no "real" bodily disease, but still complains of severe pain, a placebo may be given; a positive reaction is viewed as proof of what the medical team suspected. Unfortunately, despite the veneer of diagnosis, the real reason a placebo is used in these cases is often that the members of the team strongly dislike the patient. Distressing as this motivation may seem, it's been borne out by opinion surveys of physicians and nurses.

The Placebo Response as a Research Tool

Meanwhile, what about the use of the placebo in research? During the nineteenth and early twentieth centuries, blinded controls continued at the fringes of medical science—usually, as we saw, to discredit a remedy thought to be especially outlandish. No one then thought these trials were needed as a routine or standard tool of research on all new medications, because it was still assumed that the sole basis for establishing the efficacy of a new treatment was to have a well-trained physician openly using it and keeping careful records of what happened to the patient taking it. Even as doctors admitted in practice that the mind might be a powerful force for healing, they continued to believe that the careful, scientific physician could simply *know* whether the results of a new treatment were due to the treatment itself or to the patient's imagination. (Ironically, the first physicians routinely to use blinded controls as part of the method for "proving" new drugs were the much-maligned homeopaths in the mid–nineteenth century, nearly a hundred years before regular physicians started using the placebo control in a systematic way.)

Medicine's view of what was needed for proof that new drugs worked changed markedly in the years following World War II. The double-blind randomized controlled trial (which I mentioned briefly in chapter 1) was elevated to become the gold standard of proof of drug effectiveness, because of demands for mathematical and statistical precision, and because of increased recognition that *both* the inherent healing powers of the body and the effects of imagination could easily fool even the most careful medical observers. This form of trial is supposed to reduce all possible sources of bias, so that if a treatment is shown to work for a particular condition, one can have the greatest level of scientific confidence that it will work for all patients with that condition.

Let's review what a double-blind, randomized controlled trial really is. The trial is *randomized,* meaning that patients are assigned to the two treatment groups by a flip of the coin or some similar means, to be sure that the patients getting the drug are not sicker, or older, or more likely to have other diseases, or in any way different from the controls. The trial is *double-blind,* meaning that neither the patients nor the investigators know which patient is getting which treatment. Half the patients get a dummy or placebo, and half the patients get the drug being studied; no one involved knows which is which until the code is broken at the end of the trial.

Ted Kaptchuk, who has surveyed this history carefully, argues that the victory of the double-blind randomized trial was the result of a sort of class warfare within medicine. By the old rules which were mentioned earlier, Dr. Jones of Hoboken, or Dr. Smith of Keokuk, could assess the worthiness of a new drug treatment just as well as Dr. Bigshot of Harvard; all they had to do was try the drug on enough patients and keep careful records. By the new rules, only specially trained physicians, who knew statistics and the intricacies of experimental design, were qualified to test new treatments reliably.

But Dr. Jones and Dr. Smith did not abandon their prerogatives without a fight. The university experts needed salient reasons for persuading the majority of physicians to believe only what they learned from the new clinical trials. This meant that the university physicians now had a special incentive to magnify the placebo effect—to claim that it was so powerful, and present so often, that regular physicians simply could no longer trust their unaided clinical judgment. Thus, Dr. Henry Beecher, an experimental anesthesiologist at Harvard, became a major champion of the double-blind randomized trial and also the main exponent of "the powerful placebo," as his widely quoted 1955 paper was called. (Beecher first reported the fact that on average, one-third of subjects in the placebo group will show a positive response, a figure that we'll discuss at some length in chapter 3.)

The Placebo Response: Where Things Stand Today

The confluence of historical forces you've just read about gave rise to the peculiar status of the placebo and the placebo response in the modern medical period—as we tend to call the half-century since the end of World War II. I believe modern physicians were destined to be confused and ambivalent about the placebo effect.

On the one hand, humoral medicine had been thrown on the scrap heap; and the mechanistic view of medicine that replaced it had perhaps less room for the mind influencing the body than any other theory in medical history. It appeared that medicine in the twentieth century had made all of its great scientific strides by virtually ignoring the mind. On the other hand, these strides had led to the perceived need for double-blind randomized trials; and these trials were justified by claiming that the mind was virtually all-powerful.

In the meantime, with so many proven effective drugs now available, physicians felt increasingly little need to prescribe placebos as medical treatment; doctors who did were viewed as old-fashioned and ignorant. Yet the most famous researchers at the most famous medical schools still routinely use placebos as controls in scientific experiments. If modern physicians have trouble figuring out just what "placebo" and "placebo response" actually mean, and tend to think of these terms in a negative light, we can hardly blame them.

During the last half-century, indeed mostly in the last twenty-five years, medicine has seen a profound change in its basic ethical code. Even in earlier centuries, a few voices had been raised against the routine use of deception by physicians. In the late 1700s, the Scottish physician Dr. John Gregory spoke out in favor of medical honesty, and Richard Cabot, whom we saw discussing placebos in 1903, called attention to their use only to condemn what he called "falsehood in medicine." But Gregory's and Cabot's were minority voices. Most physicians continued to agree with Plato's view that the moral rule against lying didn't apply to physicians—as whether a person lived or died might depend on the doctor's hopeful or pessimistic words about his possible recovery.

This comfortable formula changed dramatically in the U.S. within the past twenty-five years. The current view of medical ethics is that the relationship between physician and patient should not be seen as a kind of parent-child relationship, but much more as a relationship between adults. Deceiving patients basically deprives them of all opportunity to become involved in making such medical decisions about their own care as whether or not to undergo surgery. According to the old ethic, patients should simply trust their doctors and have surgery or not as the doctor advised. The new medical ethics insists, though patients are free to ask for and follow their doctors' advice, the final decision as to what one does with one's own body ultimately rests with each individual. To be able to make such decisions, or at least be involved in the discussion, people need to know the truth about their disease, its possible outcomes, and the full range of medical options available. This is the basis for the rise of the growing "patient's rights" movement.

The new approach to medical ethics serves further to make the average physician think negatively about the idea of *placebo.* In the previous chapter, I defined "placebo response" in such a way as to remove it from any deceptive practices. To evoke a positive placebo response in the patient, you simply have to do something which alters (for the better) the symbolic significance the patient attaches to the disease or to the treatment; you don't have to lie to anyone.

My definition, a highly technical one, is not necessarily understood by many physicians today. So far as they can understand, "placebo" is still stuck back in history with Thomas Jefferson's bread pills and drops of colored water. Even Jefferson had ethical problems with those practices; in the very next line of his letter, he referred to those placebos as a "pious fraud." Yet if "placebo" means lying to the medical establishment, and ethical physicians today are not supposed to lie to patients, then we cannot blame modern doctors from looking askance at the very idea of placebo.

In the next chapter, I'll discuss how to release the placebo response from its long-time negative image. So doing will lead us to explore what, if any, personality traits encourage the placebo response and from there to the concept of the inner pharmacy—which will serve as the guiding metaphor throughout the remainder of this book.

THREE

The Placebo Response: Which of Us Is Eligible?

"I regard the placebo response as a pure example of healing elicited by the mind; far from being a nuisance, it is, potentially, the greatest therapeutic ally doctors can find in their efforts to mitigate disease. I believe further that the art of medicine is the selection of treatments and their presentation to patients in ways that increase their effectiveness through the activation of placebo responses."

—Dr. Andrew Weil

Before we begin to prove that the placebo response is a positive phenomenon, let's briefly revisit its negative image from another perspective: human nature.

Placebo Negativity and Human Nature

Human nature is replete with blind spots, envy, fear, and often irrational prejudices. Since healers are only human, it stands to reason they'd possess these personality traits. Take the following example.

Dueling Acupuncturists

An American scientist, attending an international conference on alternative medicine, observed the following scene. Among the thirty or so practitioners in the meeting room were two Koreans who met, discovered they were both acupuncturists, and began to chat amicably until the conference was called to order. All participants were then asked to introduce themselves and explain the type of healing they practiced.

Only after both Koreans made their introductions did they realize they practiced somewhat dissimilar methods of acupuncture—using slightly different techniques of needle placement and depth. Upon that revelation, their friendliness immediately vanished. Each man turned on the other, accusing his countryman of practicing a type of healing that was nothing but a placebo. It will come as no surprise that both claimed only their technique was effective in altering bodily processes.

This anecdote teaches us a number of things. First, it shows how sensitive most of us are when it comes to our beliefs about healing, and how suspicious we are of "the other": whatever kind of healing doesn't make sense according to our own beliefs.

To the conventional American M.D. practicing in the U.S., acupuncture might be "the other," which couldn't possibly be effective, since Western science denies the existence of the points and meridians upon which ancient Chinese practice of acupuncture is based. For our two Koreans, a somewhat different form of acupuncture than the one each of them preferred was "the other." To those who advocate herbal and natural remedies, the drugs prescribed by M.D.'s are "the other," since substances not found in nature but synthesized in a chemical laboratory must be harmful. When so many of us suspiciously cling to such diverse beliefs and theories, it's difficult if not impossible for us to agree about healing, perhaps especially about the placebo effect.

If we compile the placebo's entire historical track record as detailed in the last chapter, we find scientists tend to consider placebos lies or quackery when used in medical treatment, and a nuisance (even if a necessary nuisance) when used in medical research. That, as we've observed, is enough to make the placebo unpopular among the medical community. But it's not only physicians and scientists who have serious reservations about the placebo. Lay people in our society have long been troubled with processes that affect *only the mind.* We have, for example, felt mental illness is somehow less real than physical illness, and that psychiatrists are not genuine doctors in the same sense that surgeons or obstetricians are. Generally, we look down on people whose minds are "easily influenced," especially those whose bodies are then affected by the mental changes—people whom we call " hysterical" or "suggestible."

We likewise assume *we* would never get better merely by taking a placebo; if it happens to other people, it's probably also true they never had a real disease to begin with and their problem must have been "all in their heads." If the placebo is nothing more than an imaginary cure for imaginary disease, it's no wonder that the Korean acupuncturists would choose to insult each other by using the word as a slur.

We've already uncovered enough scientific clues to suspect that the placebo response is much more than "an imaginary cure for an imaginary disease." But that negative assessment leads us in turn to another puzzle question. Just what sorts of people experience a placebo response? And how are they different from other people—if they're different at all? Does the difference lie in personality traits, or in other factors?

Who Responds to Placebos?

In the 1950s and 1960s, a good deal of attention was devoted to trying to identify the so-called *placebo responder* or "placebo personality type." The impulse for this research is one we recognize today as blatantly unscientific, although scientists persisted in doing it. Basically, randomized double-blind controlled studies were a lot of trouble to perform. In effect, the scientists who had to conduct them—because of the newfound appreciation for the importance of the placebo response—took out their resentment on the subjects who demonstrated this response. The scientists reasoned: If we could only figure out in advance who these troublesome placebo responders are, we could eliminate them from the research study, and make it a lot easier to prove if the drug works or doesn't work. Then we could get quicker and more reliable experimental results with fewer subjects.

The scientists started to go down the list of constant, measurable personality variables. Do older people respond to placebos more than younger ones? Do women respond more frequently than men? How about the less educated as opposed to college graduates? Do subjects who are susceptible to hypnosis respond better to placebos as well? What about people who have more or less trust in the doctor?

At first, a number of studies seemed to turn up associations between placebo response and one or more of the above factors; yet later studies showed no association or exactly the opposite association. The virtually unanimous conclusion among those reviewing the placebo literature today is that there is no such thing as the placebo responder, if what we mean by that is some fixed, more or less permanent personality type.

Some experts would state this conclusion universally—no personality characteristics have been shown reliably to predict placebo response. But there may be an exception.

The Importance of Acquiescence

Clinical psychologists Seymour Fisher and Roger Greenberg, of the psychiatry department at the State University of New York Medical School, while concurring for the most part with this general statement, nevertheless argue that there *is* one particular personality feature which has been linked to placebo responsiveness. The studies showing this are reliable enough, and have been repeated enough times, to give us some confidence that this association is valid.

They term this feature *acquiescence*, and describe people who possess it as tending to be open, trusting, and uninhibited. This type was initially described as conformist, eager to do what everyone else seemed to expect of them. Subsequent studies showed that this was too negative a portrayal. In actuality, acquiescent individuals may be "other-people oriented": Faced with a problematic situation, they may prefer to cope in ways that involve linkages with those around them, rather than in reserved, solitary ways.

Fisher and Greenberg note that according to the psychological studies, two things seem to be true about people with high acquiescence scores. They are more likely to respond positively to placebos. And they are also more likely to respond to other medications. For Fisher and Greenberg, this finding further breaks down the supposed split between mind and body, and between the placebo response and "real" drug responses:

> ***"That acquiescence simultaneously predicts reactions to placebos and active drugs ... highlights the point ... that the boundary between 'active' drug and placebo is ambiguous. ... The usual separation of placebo response as a psychological species and drug response as a biological species is difficult to maintain because acquiescence predicts for both realms."***

The connection between what Fisher and Greenberg call acquiescence and the placebo response is vital to a concept which will be referred to frequently in later chapters: the enormous role human relationships play in evoking a positive placebo response. As already stated, acquiescent personalities tend to use relationships in a positive way when faced with life problems, becoming even more involved in relationships when under stress. These relationships then become a powerful tool in helping that person deal with her problem. (In later chapters we will see what lessons all the rest of us can learn from that coping style.)

"We Have Met the Placebo Responder, and He Is Us"

Once we get past acquiescence, however, we must conclude that the *placebo responder* is no particular personality type. But this somewhat negative finding has an important positive implication. If we look first at those things about ourselves that remain largely unchanged over time, and then examine the circumstances in which we find ourselves at one particular moment, whether or not we respond to placebos seems to be primarily determined by the situation or setting and much less by any enduring personality traits. That implies that under the right circumstances, any of us might or might not respond positively, or negatively for that matter, to a placebo. The implication that virtually none of us is inherently resistant to the placebo's influence is the attitude assumed in this book. The search for the placebo responder also produced a second positive outcome.

Anxiety Level and the Placebo Response

Yes, another variable associated with the positive placebo response did appear in a reproducible fashion: *anxiety level.* That is, the more anxious the subject, the higher the incidence of a positive response. In chapter 9 we will see that one chemical pathway which may transmit the placebo message throughout the body is the stress/relaxation pathway. If the stress pathway is "tuned" to a higher level at the start of the experiment, there is a greater chance that a stress reduction factor could facilitate a measurable change in the subject's state of health. This strongly suggests that the stress/relaxation pathway is indeed one of the chemical pathways involved in the placebo response. This suggestion does not negate the point that anyone, under the proper circumstances, can be a placebo reactor—as how anxious you are is likely to vary with the situation, rather than remain constant at all times.

The Placebo Response as Threat

To reiterate, the search for the placebo responder was an unscientific exercise, because the idea that motivated it was a scientific fallacy: assuming that experimental results would be more reliable if placebo responders could be excluded from the subject pool. Fisher and Greenberg would characterize that mindset, which attempted to eliminate placebo responders, as a mythical quest for a "biologically pure" drug.

I would argue in addition that this search for the placebo reactor-type was part and parcel of the stigma associated with placebo. If you could delineate the personality type of the placebo responder, then maybe you could show that this person is *not like you.* If you find the idea of responding to placebo embarrassing, which naturally follows from the idea that the placebo is trickery, so that the placebo responder would apparently be an especially gullible sort of person, then you naturally want to put as much distance as possible between yourself and the placebo responder.

My hope in writing this book is that you will not fall into the same trap of putting a negative connotation on the placebo response, and thus shut yourself off from the possibility that it could come to your aid when you need it. I hope you will decide that you, and I, and all of us share the potential to respond to this very powerful and positive healing influence; and that no trickery need be involved in making that happen.

The Placebo Response: When Honesty Is Key

As scientists further studied the placebo response, the next myth to go by the wayside was the linkage between the placebo response and deception. Physicians had for centuries assumed that if sugar pills worked, they could only work because the patient did not know what they really were. No one could conceive of the possibility of handing a patient sugar pills, saying, "This is a bottle of sugar pills," and still having the patient get better.

Telling Research Subjects the Truth

Two psychiatrists, Lee Park and Lino Covi, decided in the early 1960s to study truth-telling in the use of placebos. They were doing research on patients attending a psychiatric outpatient clinic; all suffered from what at the time was generally termed "neurosis." The patients had quite a number of different bodily symptoms, which were thought to be part of their condition, and Park and Covi were using a detailed symptom checklist to give each patient a numerical score to keep track of total symptoms over time. Previous patients had been given various such drugs as minor tranquilizers and treatments like psychotherapy. The authors used the symptom checklist scores to determine which treatment or set of treatments worked best at reducing symptoms. Some studies had involved placebo control groups, and as expected, a number of patients got noticeably better while taking placebos. In those studies, no subject knew whether he was receiving a placebo or the study drug.

Now Park and Covi enrolled a group of fifteen new patients in a trial with neither an "active" drug group nor psychotherapy. Instead, after the patients went through the symptom checklist process, they were given a bottle of pills. The experimenters told them frankly, "These are sugar pills, which contain no active medicine." Then they added that despite that fact, many patients had gotten better after taking one of the pills three times a day for a week. A check-up visit would be held at the end of that week of pill-taking.

When fourteen of the fifteen subjects returned a week later, the new symptom checklists showed that thirteen of those fourteen had significantly reduced symptoms. Park and Covi next did something which is sadly rare among scientists studying the placebo response. Not content merely to record numbers, they actually held conversations with their subjects, attempting to ascertain what was going on inside their heads.

From these conversations, the scientists learned, first of all, that not all their subjects had believed them about what was being prescribed. In fact, the fourteen subjects could be divided into three roughly equal groups. The first group took the scientists at their word and assumed they were taking sugar pills. The second group decided you simply couldn't trust psychiatry researchers. Although they'd been told otherwise, they believed the pills were really some kind of tranquilizer—and that they'd been lied to possibly to make the study more accurate or because there would be less chance of their getting hooked on the drug. The third group was merely unsure of what they had received.

The numbers in each group had grown too small to make valid statistical comparisons, but Park and Covi noted that the two "certain" groups—those sure they were getting sugar pills and those convinced they were getting "real" medicine—reported more substantial improvement than the "uncertain" group. Those people confident that they were getting "real" drugs also reported a number of side effects they had felt throughout the week; but no one thinking she was getting a placebo reported any side effects at all.

Park and Covi next asked the "certain-placebo" subjects how they could account for their having gotten better. Despite the limited size of the group, their answers give us some of the most important clues about what physicians must do to trigger a placebo response in their patients. About half of these subjects said that they got better because they took the placebo, while the other half claimed they improved because somehow they had drawn upon their own innate abilities to cope.

One woman reported that every time she took one of the placebos, she reminded herself that she really *could* do something to better her own condition. Some other subjects also testified they appreciated the fact that they were *not* getting an "active" drug, and so were spared the likely side effects and the risks of addiction.

By contrast, the "certain-real drug" group explained that, because they thought they were getting an active drug, they saw their symptoms improving. The improvement served to reinforce their views that the pills were genuine medicine.

One serious problem with the study—besides its limited size—should be mentioned. Park and Covi told their subjects that later on, after the placebo week, they would be getting other forms of treatment if needed. This could have meant that they were doing not so much a "nonblind placebo" study as a waiting-list study. It has been shown on a number of occasions that patients on waiting lists to receive mental health services get better at a rate faster than the natural history of their conditions would suggest—that knowing you're going to be receiving future help may be sufficient to moderate the symptoms of various mental illnesses. Thus, it's possible that Park and Covi's subjects were simply biding time, as it were, as they awaited the real treatment.

It's even possible they assumed, consciously or unconsciously, they could make the doctors happy by feeling better right away, and that, by making the doctors happy, they were assuring themselves better treatment down the road.

But it is of some interest that neither of these explanations were given by the subjects whom Park and Covi interviewed. Either we simply discount their statements as delusional, or we find credible their beliefs that some combination of taking the placebo and better appreciating their own powers of coping made a difference in their symptoms, thus demonstrating the mind-body connection.

Emotions and Wellness

That we are virtually all potential placebo receptors is good news, as is the fact that medical science is making progress on the mind-body front generally. In both conventional and alternative medicine, people are becoming much more comfortable with the ways the mind and the body can interact. Scientists are discovering new connections between the imagination and the emotions and human health and illness.

The possibility that a treatment may be good and powerful, precisely because it has its main impact on the body through the mind, is now one we can look at with a higher level of comfort and curiosity. And that sets the stage for a more positive approach to the placebo response—in keeping with the definition, based on symbolic significance, that we offered in chapter 1—as we prepare to approach the inner pharmacy.

FOUR

The Inner Pharmacy

"[I] further proclaimed that the body was God's drugstore and had in it all liquids, drugs, lubricating oils, opiates, acids and anti-acids, and every sort of drug which the wisdom of God thought necessary for human happiness and health."

—Andrew Taylor Still, 1908

As we begin to contemplate a new way of conceptualizing the placebo response, I'd like to tell you a personal anecdote that will prove extremely illustrative in our coming discussion of the inner pharmacy. The anecdote doesn't involve a life-or-death situation, but rather quality of life issues—and so, in that regard, it's much more representative of the healing matters that concern us all on a daily basis. It involves my wife, Daralyn, who is not only a gifted coauthor but an accomplished international folk dancer as well.

Daralyn's Story: The Heel Spur

In the fall of 1989, Daralyn developed a lump on her outer left heel, which she's convinced was caused by touring London in narrow-heeled shoes during a family vacation. By 1990, the lump had grown so large that practically every pair of shoes she owned hurt, especially the inflexible stage shoes Daralyn wears in her dance work. Fortunately, when she wore looser or more flexible shoes, the lump didn't hurt; still, dancing remained a problem.

When our family doctor x-rayed Daralyn's heel, he diagnosed a bony growth he called "a heel spur" (or bunion) protruding from the heelbone just under the skin surface. The orthopedic surgeon to whom Daralyn was subsequently referred told her that, because the heel spur was not likely to recede, it would have to be surgically removed. He also added that the recovery period was uncertain and her foot might be in a cast for as long as six weeks. Since Daralyn's dance company was performing monthly, and because she felt the troupe needed her despite the pain of dancing, she kept postponing the surgery.

In the autumn of 1990, Daralyn met a psychic healer named Patricia, and asked her if she could help with the heel spur. Patricia first told Daralyn to close her eyes, then guided her into a state of relaxation, addressed her soul, affirmed its divine state, and called for the restoration of physical perfection through remembrance of the body's original blueprint—all in a few minutes. After two weeks, Daralyn didn't notice any change in her condition and began to have doubts about whether psychic healing would work for her. Nevertheless, she returned to Patricia, who repeated the healing process. Following that second visit, Daralyn, who had no scheduled dance performances during this period, got busy with other things and forgot about the matter.

Perhaps a month later, we were entertaining another of Daralyn's friends who also practices alternative healing. After she left, I was massaging Daralyn's feet as we continued the discussion on healing we had begun with our visitor. Suddenly, Daralyn gasped, "Speaking of healing! Look, the lump is gone!" I examined her heel, momentarily at a loss for words—and unable to deny that the growth which had existed for more than a year had vanished, apparently very gradually, during the previous month.

A few years later, Daralyn, in the course of taking one of our children to the family doctor, mentioned to him how the heel spur had simply disappeared without surgery but apparently through psychic intervention. He smiled and answered, "Well, if it worked, it's just fine."

For whatever reason, Daralyn's spur has been gone for nine years and has never shown signs of returning.

Daralyn's story—however we interpret it—provides some genuinely eye-opening clues to what we've learned so far about the *science* of the placebo response. I'm going to put on my scientist's hat to ask: Assuming that the heel spur went away (which I certainly cannot deny), what would explain the healing? How could I, as a scientific physician, account for it?

One possible explanation is that psychic healing works. Western medical science has no idea how it could work, and I don't know of any scientific proof that it does work, but, as a medical scientist, I would have to remain open to the possibility. There's a saying among scientists, "Just because you have no proof that something works, doesn't mean that you *do* have proof that it *doesn't* work." The question has to remain open, at least until more research is done.

Another possible explanation is that the heel spur did get better on its own. A common misconception is that bone is dead and inert. We think so because we virtually never see live bone; the bone we have always come in contact with (such as a skeleton hanging in a science classroom) is necessarily dead bone. But live bone is one of the most dynamic tissues in the body. New bits of bone are always being manufactured and old bits are always being absorbed. A heel spur or bunion or similar bony overgrowth is usually a response to some localized pressure on the bone. When the pressure goes away, it may take a while, but eventually the body might be expected to absorb the no-longer-needed bone.

The explanation, "It got better on its own," which we've already touched on, is very important to keep in mind. In chapter 10, we'll see that this factor—the natural history of the disease—is one of the most important *mimics* of the true placebo response, for which careful scientists need to watch out. Is this a plausible explanation in Daralyn's case? One factor that goes strongly against the "natural history" explanation is that two experienced physicians thought that the heel spur had lasted too long to go away on its own. One of these physicians, our family doctor, was by his philosophy inclined to recommend that surgery be avoided or postponed if at all possible.

Finally there is a third explanation. Did Daralyn's state of mind have anything to do with the cure? She consciously believes that she harbored reservations about the psychic healing and had in fact put it out of her mind. But she did go back to the healer a second time—unlike the family doctor or the surgeon—which may mean that, because of her initial reservations about faith healing, it took two sessions for the "faith" to take root. Subconsciously, she may have harbored more "underground" faith, or hope, or expectation in the process than she realized. Could such mental forces have had any influence on what happened in her body? I deeply believe they could, and in this chapter I'll tell you how and why.

Inner Healing: Our Gift to Ourselves

The human body is a genuinely marvelous creation, and one of its most impressive features is the variety of built-in treatments for most of the disorders that might afflict it. The body can be made ill by germs, but it contains an immune system which does battle with and eventually rids itself of the germs. It could be poisoned by certain chemicals, but the stomach might well reject such toxins from the body. Even without any medical care at all, many people are healthy a good deal of the time and can live fairly long lives.

Let's suppose that we have studied these inner health-restorers and now know a good deal about how they work. When the body is ill or in pain, some of its chemical substances are automatically produced in greater quantity than normal and may then eliminate the sickness or discomfort. We could think of this set of health-restoring features as *the body's inner pharmacy*. When a person is sick, and then gets better as time passes, we could explain the change by saying that the body's inner pharmacy has been at work.

Now, suppose we discover that this inner pharmacy doesn't merely respond according to an inherent sense of the body's internal state.

Suppose that environmental factors can affect the way the pharmacy operates. Suppose we realize that there are things we can do—and that others can do for us—that awaken our inner pharmacy, causing it to respond more promptly and more efficiently to various illnesses. That means we can, in effect, phone in a prescription to our own inner pharmacy. Suppose the signals that turn on or turn up the inner pharmacy are themselves very safe, so we need not be concerned they'll make us sicker.

The inner pharmacy then becomes a metaphor to assist us in thinking about the placebo response. This metaphor sheds new light on the nineteenth-century debate about how cures were produced by placebos. Recall that physicians disagreed as to whether they were seeing cures produced by the healing power of the imagination, the natural history of the disease, or the body's inherent healing powers. Notice that, according to the metaphor of the inner pharmacy, there is really very little difference between the healing power of the imagination and the body's inherent healing powers.

As I will argue when we come to look at modern neuroscience in chapter 9, the human body is hard-wired to translate the imagination (and other symbolic signals) into natural healing forces. I have taken the term "hard-wired" from computer jargon to emphasize the difference between the equipment—or hardware—and software. You can install new software, which will instruct the computer how to perform a function such as bookkeeping. You could later erase all the software files (either deliberately or accidentally), and then the computer would no longer be able to perform that function. If the function is hard-wired, it's built in as part of the basic design; you can't erase it as long as the computer is intact.

The inner pharmacy is hard-wired to be one of the body's inherent healing powers. If we imagine that, when we were born, we purchased our bodies at a dealership, the inner pharmacy wasn't an option; it was standard equipment.

Still, while there may not really be much difference between the placebo response and self-healing or spontaneous recovery, there is some.

Spontaneous Healing and the Placebo Response: How They Differ

It may be that the very same body processes and chemicals operate in the placebo response and in self-healing or spontaneous recovery. In spontaneous recovery, the body goes about its business unaided; no message from our own minds or from other persons' minds comes to stimulate the process. In the placebo response, we presume that a message has made an impact on the mind, which then turns on new chemical pathways, or at least accentuates and strengthens the pathways that are already operating. So there's a measurable difference in outcome between the placebo responder and the spontaneous healer.

For those opposed to medicine of any kind on the basis of "unnaturalness," it is important to remember that there is nothing unnatural or artificial about the body's inner pharmacy, as we are using the metaphor. It's part of the built-in, fully natural healing power with which all of us were originally designed.

In fact, it's ironic that a healer strongly opposed to the idea of getting treatment from chemicals may have originated the metaphor of the inner pharmacy. As you'll recall from the beginning of this chapter, Dr. Andrew Taylor Still, the founder of osteopathy, described the human body as "God's drugstore." Indeed, by listing opiates in "God's drugstore," he was being quite prescient: Not for another half-century did scientists discover opium-like chemicals called *endorphins* produced by the human body's inner pharmacy (as we'll see in chapter 9).

Now let's take note of something very central to the body's inner pharmacy. There's no rule that says you have to choose between the internal and the external. The body is fully capable of responding to outside substances or processes which can promote healing. For most illnesses, the fastest and most complete healing will occur when we combine the actions of the outside healing processes with the work of the body's inner pharmacy.

There's a popular newspaper cartoon that reads, "If I can't have the real medicine, then I want the very best placebo." The only kind of physician who would offer us this choice is one not truly interested in healing. There is no reason we cannot have *both* the real medicine and the very best placebo. And there is no reason why real medicine cannot itself be the very best placebo, if it sends the right symbolic signals to our inner pharmacy.

Let's go one image further as we visualize the body's inner pharmacy. Picture the pharmacy as an intersection or meeting place, where practitioners and devotees of all types of healing can at last feel comfortable together. M.D.'s, osteopaths, chiropractors, aromatherapists, acupuncturists, faith healers, and all other sorts of healers (and healees) can congregate there. As we've seen, they disagree about many things, but what they can all agree on is that each of their types of healing is capable of sending symbolic messages to those patients who have the proper mental viewpoint for stimulating the inner pharmacy. Each sort of healing practitioner can agree that the inner pharmacy is a great ally to them in their healing quest. Indeed, some of the healers might admit that all their treatments really do is turn on and strengthen the inner pharmacy in a particularly effective way for a certain group of sufferers. Other healers will still insist that they offer some processes which are separate from what the inner pharmacy does. But all of them respect the inner pharmacy and agree that their work would be much harder, and much less successful, without it. In fact, a particularly helpful aspect of the inner pharmacy is that it directs attention away from the healer and her treatments and focuses on the person who is ill.

The Patient as Healer

Our "acquiescence" friends Fisher and Greenberg observe that the tendency in conventional medicine, and in any healing system to some degree, is to attribute cures to the skill and power of the healer, ignoring any possible contribution by the patient's own resources. (As we will see in chapter 11, alternative medicine may tend to do this less, which may be one of the reasons for its popularity today.) Stigmatizing the placebo responder as "passive," they suggest, may be missing the boat:

"The fact that individuals can take advantage of cues and ideas offered by the placebo context is not a sign of passivity but rather of the ability to mobilize oneself imaginatively. What is called passivity may really be a willingness to be receptive to communications."

If we use the metaphor of the inner pharmacy, we'll be much less likely to forget the important contribution that each of us makes to our own healing processes.

The inner pharmacy as a metaphor of the placebo response leads, I feel, to a much more wholesome and positive picture of the role of the placebo response in human healing. In the rest of the book, I'll be showing you evidence that suggests this picture is reasonably realistic, and what it signifies for various healing practices.

There are two more medical matters related to the placebo response we should be clear about.

Uncertainty and Variability in the Placebo Response

Uncertainty is the one aspect of the placebo response that could legitimately lead to a negative view of it among medical scientists, especially those who discount or ignore the vital role of the inner pharmacy in the healing process. Scientists, after all, like events that can be predicted with lawlike regularity, but the placebo response has always refused to cooperate with them. What turns on my inner pharmacy may not turn on yours; or what turns on mine in one situation may fail to do so in another situation; or what turns mine on full blast one time, may turn it on only a little on another occasion.

You'll recall that early work on the placebo suggested, on average, approximately one-third of subjects would have a positive placebo response. Still, as we saw, there is no predicting by personality characteristics who those affected will be. If the reaction to the situation, rather than enduring personality traits, is what determines the placebo response, then no one has yet found a way to measure exactly of what that situational reaction consists. Predicting who will respond to placebo and who won't remains an inherently uncertain business.

It's even a bit more complicated than that. By now we know that the one-third figure for the average placebo response has been repeated over and over in the medical literature—as if to say, "All right, we cannot be certain about who exactly will respond as an individual; but at least we can be fairly certain about the overall size and scope of the response." It turns out that this sense of certainty is misleading as well, as the following anecdote indicates.

Drugs for Ulcers: What Dan Moerman Found

Anthropologists usually don't carry out placebo-controlled studies of new drugs. Daniel Moerman of the University of Michigan at Dearborn, around 1980, was interested in the interaction between drugs and culture, especially in how the various medicinal plants used by Native Americans might have worked. The anthropologist found that he could read the medical journals just as well as anyone else; so, if medical investigators wanted to do studies comparing drugs with placebos, Moerman could read them and do what he wanted with the results.

Moerman, as it turned out, had an original and clever idea. The usual randomized, double-blind, placebo-controlled study is designed for one purpose only: to demonstrate whether or not the experimental drug causes patients to get better. What happens to the subjects in the placebo group, and why, is of no interest. The difference between the placebo group and the drug group (or *arm*, as scientists term it) is all that counts.

To understand the placebo response in a scientific sense, one has to give the same placebo but under different conditions, to see if the conditions alter how the placebo works. That means there needs somehow to be an experimental and a control group, but both have to get placebos.

What Moerman observed was that as long as only one or two studies were done comparing any single drug to placebo, you could never find out anything interesting about how the placebos worked. But suppose ten or twenty or even thirty studies were done, each comparing the same active drug to placebo, and measuring exactly the same symptom or disease process. It would be even better if the measurement were of something quantifiable and objective, so that you could be more confident in making comparisons among the studies. Then, by comparing what happened in the placebo arms of all of these studies, you could perhaps discern patterns which would provide clues about the placebo response. And so Moerman went searching through the medical journals, and finally found what he wanted.

In the mid–1970s, the emergence of a new drug, cimetidine (Tagamet), revolutionized the treatment of ulcers. Physicians had always assumed that ulcers were related to an excess of acid in the stomach and the first part of the small intestine, but previously, all they could do was give antacids to neutralize the acid once it formed. Cimetidine was the first of a totally new class of drugs that had the power to turn off the acid at its source. There was great excitement about it, and scientists all over the world began subjecting cimetidine to controlled studies.

Moerman was able eventually to research a total of thirty-one studies that compared cimetidine to placebo in a randomized, double-blind fashion. Moreover, each study had virtually the same design: Physicians first looked into the patient's stomach with a flexible scope passed through the mouth, which displayed that an ulcer was there and how big it was. One month later, all subjects were rescoped to determine if the ulcer had shrunk or healed completely.

Laying the thirty-one studies side by side, Moerman noted there was a very close and uniform clustering of the success rates of the cimetidine arm of all the studies, roughly around 70 to 75 percent healing at one month. Whatever way cimetidine performed inside the body seemed to be quite unaffected by other environmental factors. But here was a puzzle: The studies did not uniformly show that cimetidine was better than placebo. Indeed, about half the studies concluded that cimetidine was better than placebo, and the other half that it wasn't.

The solution to the puzzle, Moerman eventually discovered, had nothing to do with cimetidine whatever—but everything to do with placebo. The placebo response *on average* was about one third of the ulcers healing at the end of the month. That turned out to be almost identical to the response rate that Henry Beecher had reported in his review of pain studies in 1955, and which scientists had consistently reported ever since.

What Moerman could now see clearly was that this "average" masked a tremendous variation. The placebo-arm cure rates in his thirty-one studies ranged all over the landscape. There was a low study in which only 10 percent of ulcers were healed after a month of placebos; and a high study in which there was a 90 percent placebo cure rate; and just about everything in between. And here lay the solution to the puzzle, for it turned out that when the placebo effect was at the high end of the spectrum, the studies could not show any statistical difference between cimetidine and placebo; but at the low end of the placebo-response spectrum, cimetidine easily emerged the winner. It was the placebo response rate and not the cimetidine response rate that determined the overall results of the study.

Moerman, as an anthropologist, was interested in whether cultural differences alter the likelihood that a given signal will turn on our inner pharmacies. So he went on and classified the studies by country in which the research was done. While this part of his conclusion was more tentative, he showed some trends of national differences in placebo response rate. Some of the studies with the lowest placebo healing, for instance, were done in Denmark, while some of the highest placebo response rates occurred in German studies.

All the scientists doing these studies cared about cimetidine and not about the placebo response. So their papers did not report anything about the emotional environment in which the studies were conducted, and certainly no one interviewed the subjects, as Park and Covi had done, to see what was on their minds. We can only speculate what might have made the differences that resulted in such widely varying placebo responses.

However, two comments could be added here. We've seen that the natural history of the illness is one of the alternative explanations for a "cure" that might otherwise be attributed to the placebo response: Ulcers either heal because they are treated with cimetidine, or they heal because of the body's own natural recuperative processes. We don't have to add any "signals" from the external environment, or emotions, or expectations, to explain what happens. (We'll look at some of these skeptical arguments in detail in chapter 10.)

This explanation makes sense if we look only at the averages, for it's logical that about a third of ulcers might heal on their own after a month. That, taken by itself, would eliminate the so-called placebo response.

If we look at the ranges as opposed to the averages, the explanation is much harder to accept. Why would it be that, in some clinics, only 10 percent of ulcers heal by themselves at the end of one month, while in another clinic in another country, 80 percent do? Suggesting that there is such a wide variation in the natural history of ulcer disease is almost to admit that we don't understand very much about what causes or cures ulcers. At any rate, it is just as thorny to explain such a wide variation in natural history as to demonstrate why a placebo effect should occur, especially when you add the fact that stomach acid levels have been known for a long time to be altered by emotional factors.

To sum up: It is often the case that skeptical scientists and physicians dismiss the importance of the placebo response because it is, by its nature, so unpredictable. Roughly a third of patients in research studies will show a placebo response, but we cannot tell who they are, and an individual who responds to placebo in one double-blind study might not in another. When the placebo response rate runs from 10 to 90 percent, many would simply throw up their hands. Maybe it's real, but what's its value? How can you study it scientifically? We might as well just forget about it and study the definitive laws of biochemistry and physiology.

This argument really uses a double standard when you keep in mind cimetidine healed about 70 to 75 percent of ulcers. And exactly the same things we said about placebo could be said about cimetidine—only to a lesser degree. We have, in fact, no idea what was different about the 25 to 30 percent of people who did not respond to cimetidine. We can claim that they had drug resistance, or that they metabolized the drug differently. Still, unless we have genuine biochemical evidence to explain those hypotheses, all we are really saying is, "They didn't get better and we don't know why." According to a modern theory of ulcers which has arisen since Moerman's work, the 25 to 30 percent may have failed to heal because their stomachs were infected with the bacteria *Helicobacter pylorii.* Studies of various drug combinations to get rid of *Helicobacter pylorii* show that the drugs eliminate the bacteria in maybe 90 to 95 percent of patients; and we have the same problem explaining why the other 5 to 10 percent don't get rid of the bacteria. And many people have the bacteria in their stomachs, yet do not get ulcers.

Since there is no drug that works 100 percent of the time or is 100 percent predictable, we should not use variability in the placebo response to discount it or to imagine that we cannot come to better understand it and the metaphor of the inner pharmacy. The variability does leave us with an element of mystery. In the epilogue I'll come back to the question of mystery and claim that it's an irreducible element of the placebo response and the workings of the inner pharmacy.

So far, we've introduced and defined the placebo response, looked at its history, questioned which of us are most receptive to it, and introduced the metaphor of the inner pharmacy to view it in an appropriately positive light. In the next five chapters we'll review in more detail further evidence and pertinent theories of how the enigmatic placebo response actually works.

FIVE

The Placebo Response and Expectancy

"A case was related by the late Dr. Gregory, in which a patient who had taken twenty-five drops of laudanum, thinking it was a purgative, was disturbed all night by the evacuations from his bowels. [Laudanum contains opium, which is notorious for causing severe constipation.]"

—*The Lancet*, 1836

As we learned in chapter 3, most personality traits, with the exception of acquiescence and anxiety level, failed to work as predictors of the placebo response. Still, physicians and scientists of the modern era have tried to make sense of the placebo response by asking, "How can we predict when patients or experimental subjects will react to placebo; and what sort of reaction will occur?" This chapter and the next deal in depth with two popular theories, to which you've already been briefly introduced: *expectancy* theory and *conditioning* theory.

We'll see that each theory provides clues as to which treatment techniques might enhance the workings of the inner pharmacy. We'll also note they both can predict experimental findings about the placebo response, and that they overlap and complement each other in important ways. First, here's how they differ: Expectancy theory asks, "How does what I think is going to happen in the future affect my inner pharmacy?" while conditioning theory questions, "How does what has happened to me in the past affect my inner pharmacy?"

Now let's look in detail at expectancy, beginning with this remarkable case study:

Tom, The Placebo Receptor

Dr. Stewart Wolf was one of the pioneering group of late 1940s researchers who became intrigued with the placebo response and sought to determine more about its mechanisms. Wolf at the time was studying how the function of the stomach correlated to the symptoms his research subjects reported when given various medications. His system consisted of placing a pressure-measuring tube into the stomachs of his subjects so that he could graph the actual wave forms of the movements of the stomach muscles. When his subjects reported nausea, he could clearly see a disturbed wave pattern; when they reported relief of nausea, he could see the pattern return to normal.

Wolf had given his subjects two drugs: ipecac, which causes vomiting, and atropine, which soothes the stomach and produces a peaceful muscle pattern. He next decided to see what happened when he gave the subjects sugar pills but told them that the pills were either ipecac or atropine. As he expected, many of the subjects given the dummy ipecac reported severe nausea, and many of those given the so-called atropine reported that their nausea had substantially diminished. The reactions went beyond the verbal reports: Wolf watched the stomach wave patterns and saw exactly the same changes as with the active drugs.

One subject in his laboratory, a man he called Tom, seemed especially prone to placebo responses, so Wolf decided to go the next step with him. Instead of giving him placebos for the next round of trials, Wolf gave Tom atropine and ipecac—only this time, he told him he was giving him ipecac when he was actually giving him atropine, and vice versa. Tom reported that he was experiencing severe nausea after he had taken the "ipecac," which was really atropine, and his stomach tracings showed the nausea pattern. When given the "atropine," (which was now really the ipecac) and told that it should soothe his stomach, Tom shortly afterward reported relief; and his stomach tracings indeed returned to a normal pattern.

That's expectancy in a nutshell. Now we're going to examine it to a fuller extent.

Expectancy Theory

On one level, this theory is quite simple. It proposes that if you count on improving after you receive a medicine, there's a good chance that you will—even if the improvement cannot be explained by any of the chemical components of the medication. That indicates that the mental state of expectancy, by itself, can have an impact on the state of health or illness of the rest of the body. A person's expectation can produce a bodily effect under many different circumstances, and not merely when the person is given a substance that is chemically inactive.

Stewart Wolf's studies have had a major influence on ensuing placebo research for several reasons. He was one of the first researchers to show that the placebo response exceeded a person's subjective impression. Previous work on pain, for instance, had to rely solely on the subject's report. Because there is no objective measurement for pain, scientists have no way of knowing how much discomfort you are suffering except by asking you. That had led most physicians to assume that placebo responses were not "real" in a bodily sense. A sugar pill might make you think you were better, but it could not possibly have any effect on the body itself. Wolf blasted this myth, which was based on the old assumption of the mind-body split, by showing that placebos had as much effect on objectively measurable bodily processes as on the subjects' verbal reports.

Wolf went beyond even that by showing how powerful the placebo effect might be, at least in selected patients like Tom. The second medical myth he disproved was that even if a patient might occasionally respond to a placebo, the effect could never be as strong or as long-lasting as a response to a "real" drug. The case of Tom would seem to put that misconception to rest.

The following anecdotes illustrate still other aspects of expectancy theory and show why it has been so widely adopted by investigators.

Can the Placebo Response Reverse the Chemical Power of a Drug?

In 1970, Wolf's findings were taken a step further by Dr. Thomas Luparello and colleagues in the Department of Psychiatry at the Downstate Medical Center in Brooklyn, New York. Dr. Luparello's team recruited twenty patients who had been diagnosed with asthma, then exposed them to two drugs. One, isoproterenol, is commonly used in the treatment of asthma to expand the bronchial tubes of the lung, allowing air to flow where breathing had previously been obstructed. The other medication, carbachol, is a bronchoconstrictor and has exactly the opposite effect. Asthma would be expected to worsen when that substance is inhaled. After the subjects inhaled the drugs, the investigators measured air flow and lung volumes. Both drugs were given under two sets of conditions: one in which the subjects were told beforehand what the drug was; and the other in which the subjects were told beforehand that it was the other drug.

Each drug worked better on average when the subjects *expected* its effects. That is, when told they were getting isoproterenol and were actually being given isoproterenol, the subjects showed more flow of air into the lungs than when they took isoproterenol, believing it was carbachol. When informed they would be taking carbachol and then actually got it, their lung flow worsened more intensely than when they were told they were taking isoproterenol but actually got carbachol.

Of special interest here is what happened when four subjects given isoproterenol and five subjects given carbachol were told they were getting the other drug. The four subjects who got isoproterenol but thought it was carbachol showed an actual worsening of air flow in their lungs—consistent with the drug effect they expected, yet absolutely inconsistent with the effect produced by the chemical substance they inhaled. Five of the subjects who inhaled carbachol thinking it was isoproterenol showed an improvement in air flow—again demonstrating that the force of mental expectancy could overcome and reverse chemical effect. With a single exception, the four subjects who had the paradoxical response to isoproterenol were different from the five who had the paradoxical response to carbachol.

A final experiment of this type was performed by Drs. Yujiro Ikemi and Shunji Nakagawa in Japan. The lacquer or wax tree in Japan is much like poison ivy in the U.S., commonly producing severe allergic skin reactions in those who touch the leaves. Drs. Ikemi and Nakagawa selected fifty-seven high school students, blindfolded them, and touched them on one arm with leaves from the lacquer tree, while they brushed the other arm with leaves from the harmless chestnut tree. The experimenters told all the boys that the opposite leaf was being used respectively on each arm. In more than half the cases, the boys immediately began to show a red, itchy rash at the site that had been touched by the chestnut leaves, and no reaction at all where touched with the lacquer leaves. This happened, in many cases, despite the fact that these boys had had previous, severe reactions to the lacquer leaves and so seemed presensitized.

In some studies, expectancy effects have been so strong that the same drug acted in totally different ways, depending upon whether or not the subject had been told what it was. One study comparing the effects of chloral hydrate (a potent sleeping pill) and amphetamine (a potent "upper") showed that the two drugs acted as predicted so long as the subjects knew which ones they were getting. When the subjects did not know, the effects of the two drugs were indistinguishable.

Now here's another surprising example of expectancy theory at work.

Surgery for Coronary Disease

As has been noted, medical science was advancing rapidly after World War II, producing what seemed to be virtually numberless new cures for fatal and serious diseases. Both the public and the medical profession assumed whenever they read of a new breakthrough that the results were due solely to our better scientific understanding of how the body works, and the application of that new knowledge to diseases. No one thought that mental influences or suggestion could possibly be playing a role in any of these advances, but they were about to be proven wrong.

One of the great postwar "breakthroughs" was surgery for angina due to coronary artery disease. This was well before the modern era of coronary bypass surgery, since most surgery directly on the heart and its vessels was technically impossible in the 1940s and early 1950s. Surgeons tried to think of other ways to get more blood to flow through the coronary arteries and to relieve the severe and sometimes fatal chest pains that resulted from lack of oxygen to the heart muscle. They hit upon the idea that the mammary arteries in the chest, which served no vital function, might be diverting just enough blood away from the coronary arteries to account for the reduced flow. If they did surgery into the chest wall, in order to tie off (ligate) the mammary arteries, they could possibly make more blood flow through the coronary arteries and so relieve angina.

To test this idea, the surgeons did what surgeons have done for centuries, and still often do today: They tried the new procedure on patients with severe angina, secure in the belief that if the angina got better, they would *know* that the surgery must have been successful.

And it worked marvelously well. A substantial number of patients who received the mammary artery ligation reported that they had major reductions in angina, and could walk much longer distances, climb more stairs, and generally be much more active without having the crushing chest pain they had previously experienced. These effects seemed to last at least for many months. At first, it seemed that this relatively minor surgery was going to be the miracle cure for angina.

Then a few skeptical, and brave, surgeons began to have doubts about the procedure. They took advantage of the lax ethical standards of the day and didn't tell their subjects the truth about what was being done to them. Operations were performed on a number of patients in the same fashion that mammary artery ligation had always been performed, with one exception: They did not tighten the stitch placed around the mammary artery. The patients, waking up, had scars on their chests and pain from the incision, and thought that they had had the regular surgery; but in truth just as much blood was flowing through their mammary arteries as before. Yet these placebo-surgery patients reported almost exactly the same spectacular results as the previous patients, in terms of pain relief, increased exercise ability, and length of improvement. And just as many of them—two-thirds or more—seemed to get good results as in the "real" surgery group.

At a minimum, these pioneering controlled trials of surgery for angina showed that if mammary artery ligation worked, it did not work because it somehow shifted blood flow back toward the coronary arteries. Most observers believed that what they had seen here was a true placebo effect. Since surgery is seen by most of us as a much more powerful treatment than simply taking a pill, the placebo response observed in these patients was much more powerful than the response seen from taking most placebo pills. More patients had a response; the angina was reduced to a much greater extent; and the effects were quite long lasting. It seemed that the more powerful and more arresting the message sent to the body's inner pharmacy from the outside environment, the better that pharmacy might react.

Experience with treatments like mammary artery ligation have provided scientists with one of the most important measures of the power of expectancy. Recently, psychologist Alan Roberts and his colleagues selected five treatments for review in this manner. The treatments were originally introduced with much fanfare and promise, but all five have subsequently been rejected as a result of double-blind randomized trials showing that they do not work any better than placebo. Roberts's group focused on the early studies done with each treatment, generally without a control group. In these studies, they reasoned, the expectancy of both investigators and patients that the new treatment would work would have been at its maximum. Combining all the early, positive studies for the five treatments, Roberts saw that the outcomes had been classified as 40 percent excellent; 30 percent good; and 30 percent poor. No fewer than 70 percent of the subjects in these early trials had had either excellent or good outcomes from the use of treatments now universally believed to be worthless. According to Roberts, only a very strong therapeutic power of expectancy could explain these numbers.

One more insight was gained from the history of mammary artery surgery for angina. Another common myth about the placebo response is that though it might mimic the effects of "real" drugs or surgery, the relief it provides will of necessity be temporary, while "real" effects would be expected to be long lasting. Here again, the benefits those first subjects obtained from the sham surgery often lasted for months or years.

Another lesson taught by the mammary-artery example is the importance of a placebo control that truly mimics the "real" treatment. Seymour Fisher and Roger Greenberg emphasize this in their review of research on antidepressant medicines. Most antidepressants cause noticeable side effects (like dry mouth) in almost all patients who take them. The vast majority of research studies comparing antidepressants to placebos show that the antidepressant is better. But only a few studies have been done using an *active placebo*—that is, a dummy that mimics the same side effects as the antidepressant, only without any chemical in it that scientists think is useful in treating depression. In the studies where the side effects are the same, so subjects truly do not know which treatment they are getting, it's much more difficult to prove any superiority of antidepressants over placebo.

Since the mammary-artery experiments were carried out in those earlier days of lax ethical protections for research subjects, most physicians in the 1990s simply assumed that tests using sham surgery were a thing of the past. After all, in today's climate of fully informed consent, no patient would ever agree to be part of a study in which there was a chance of getting sham surgery. Or would they?

Arthroscopic Expectations

There was considerable interest when Dr. J. Bruce Moseley's team from the Veterans Administration Hospital at Baylor University reported in 1996 that they had carried out a placebo-controlled trial of a common surgical procedure (arthroscopy) for degenerative arthritis of the knee.

Three groups participated in the experiment: a full arthoscopy group, in which the cartilage was looked at and scraped down; a group that had the scope put into the joint and a water flush for the usual time of the surgery, but no scraping; and a group that had no surgery at all but only nicks on the skin. All subjects were told in advance the full truth about the experimental plan, and informed they wouldn't know which group they were in; yet all gave their voluntary consent. The findings were about the same as in the mammary artery experiments: no significant difference in outcome among the three groups.

The two stories we have just reviewed—the obvious success of sham surgery in curing angina in the 1950s, coupled with the experience in doing completely ethical sham-surgery experiments in the 1990s—make strong cases for the expectancy theory. In the period from the 1950s to the 1990s, medical opinion was changing, too. After reading the early work of Wolf, Park and Covi, and others, most physicians began to see that the placebo response had a lot to do with the patients' *expectations of cure.* Somehow, thinking that one is going to get better seems to be a form of mental signal that can turn on the body's inner pharmacy. But few physicians imagined that their own expectations could be equally powerful, when they were not even disclosed to the patient.

The Drugs and the Doctors' Expectations

That's what Dr. E. H. Uhlenhuth and his colleagues at the Johns Hopkins University Department of Psychiatry had to deal with when they sat down to analyze the data from a double-blind randomized study of two tranquilizers compared to placebo for psychiatric clinic patients with anxiety. These tranquilizers are generally viewed as effective for anxiety symptoms, and so the investigators naturally expected to show that in their study the tranquilizer groups did better than the placebo group. When their data did not show this, they suspected that something was wrong. After they looked more closely, it occurred to them to analyze the data according to which of two psychiatrists the patients had seen when they were being given their capsules.

According to the study protocol, the psychiatrists were supposed to treat all patients identically, and they claimed to have done so. But when they broke down the data, it turned out that if you considered only the half of the patients who had seen psychiatrist A, there was no difference between either of the tranquilizers and the placebo. If you considered only those patients seeing psychiatrist B, one of the drugs (meprobamate) was better than placebo. When the data were combined, the lack of effect on the A side obscured the effect on the B side so that overall there was no statistical difference between the medication and the control groups.

Dr. Uhlenhuth next talked in more detail to Drs. A and B. It turned out that Dr. A was a younger physician who seemed rather noncommittal to the patients, and in his own mind doubted that any of the drugs actually made a difference. Dr. B, by contrast, was older and appeared more fatherly to the patients; his own thinking was that meprobamate was definitely superior to placebo, though he was not so convinced about the other "active" drug.

Neither A nor B was consciously aware of having transmitted his personal views to any of the experimental subjects. The experiment was designed in such a way that it would have been very hard for them to do so. We can only speculate what sorts of signals A and B could have transmitted to their patients' inner pharmacies. Whatever it was, the experimental results were virtually identical to the unexpressed expectations of the two psychiatrists.

As you can see from these research findings, there seems to be a consistent thread of "mind over matter"—the ability of the body to undergo a healing change because the mind expects it to happen. In the case of the Uhlenhuth experiment, the expectancy lay perhaps more in the mind of the physician than in that of the patient, but it still worked. One case report showed a small child to be affected by the healing expectations of the parent. In one older study, patients improved more on placebos than on tranquilizers, when the medicine was administered by nurses who strongly disapproved of giving "drugs" to these patients.

Other bits of data that seem to support expectancy theory are findings about which placebos work most effectively, and for what conditions. Many investigators have found that capsules tend to work better than tablets; that injections tend to work better than drugs taken by mouth; and that injections that sting work better than painless injections. We've seen already that surgery can be an especially powerful placebo stimulus. Placebos taken four times a day seem to be more effective than placebos taken twice a day. When placebos (or drugs, for that matter) are in the form of colored capsules or coated tablets, blue, green, and purple ones seem to work especially well as sedatives and sleeping pills, while red, yellow, and orange seem to work best as stimulants or energy-boosters. All of these effects seem to go along with the natural expectancy of the average person. One patient, unlike the average person, became 100 percent convinced that his two-colored capsules would not work unless he swallowed them green end first. Needless to say, what he expected ended up happening.

Now let's discuss another vital aspect of the placebo response and expectancy theory.

Top-Down, Bottom-Up: A General Expectancy Theory of the Placebo Response

Psychologists add depth to the expectancy theory by tying it to an evolutionary view of human behavior. According to this view, the body's reaction to a message from the outside world will be a combination of two factors: the "bottom-up" processing of the incoming information, in which the higher centers of the brain analyze the new information in detail; and a "top-down" response, in which the brain quickly scans its existing inventory of behavior patterns for something that seems to match the overall pattern of the new information. The bottom-up process may take a long time, and so the human body, according to this psychological view, is hardwired to respond to some situations from the top-down reaction—a sort of "shoot first, ask questions later" mode. The top-down process is most likely to be triggered in situations where the mind-body unit regards itself as being in significant danger, and where the extra time required for a full bottom-up analysis might be too risky.

Here's an example of the two reactions at work. You see something in the grass at your feet that might be a snake. The top-down reaction is basically, "Snake!" and produces a rapid jump backward, as well as stress responses such as faster heart rate, increased blood pressure, and higher muscle tone. The bottom-up reaction is, "Let's look at this more carefully. It's long and thin and brown so it could be a snake. But it's not moving, and it's pretty straight. . . . Maybe it's actually a stick. Let me reach down carefully and touch it—yup, it's a stick." The evolutionary part of the theory proposes that for most of its history, the human race had a much better survival chance if the top-down response was the first to kick in. So natural selection favored our minds' developing and retaining a number of top-down response patterns.

The placebo response, according to expectancy theory, might be just such a top-down reaction. Since illness is a threat to the organism, the brain may well have stored in its memory files certain pathways of healing: signals that can be sent to the inner pharmacy to stimulate the release of healing chemicals. If a message is then received that resembles in its outward form something that the person *expects* to be associated with healing, that might be enough to trigger one of the stored top-down reaction pathways, leading to a release from the inner pharmacy, followed by bodily healing. That can occur even if a more careful analysis would have shown that the message was a fraud—that the pill was a sugar pill and not a chemically powerful substance.

Indeed, Dr. Herbert Benson—pioneering author of *The Relaxation Response* and a strong proponent of the placebo response—has argued that this top-down response pattern is the basic model for the placebo response. Based on that conclusion he has suggested that we replace the term "placebo response" with "remembered wellness," which Benson feels has none of the placebo's negative connotations and is a better description of what the brain actually does in calling up from its stored files one of the top-down healing responses.

To me, on the other hand, the concept of the inner pharmacy can

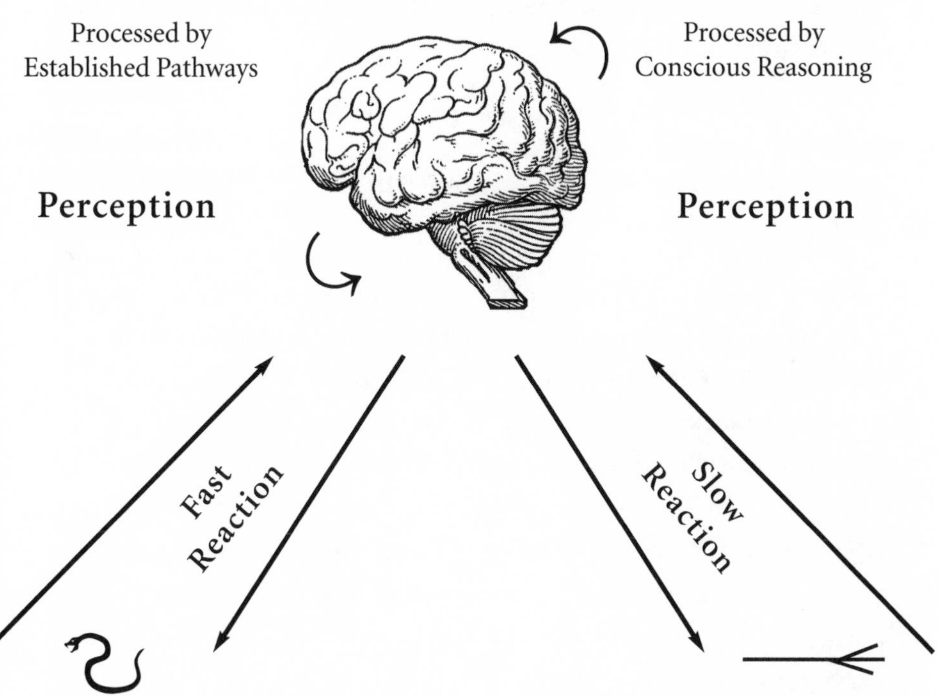

A GENERAL MODEL OF EXPECTANCY AS "TOP-DOWN" BEHAVIOR

The left-hand side of the diagram depicts *top-down* behavior. The body perceives a possible threat in the environment, and the information is processed rapidly by lower portions of the brain, using brain-behavior circuits previously laid down for automatic responses. If the environmental stimulus represents a true threat, this allows the body to rapidly mobilize threat-reducing behavior that has worked in the past.

The right-hand side of the diagram depicts *bottom-up* behavior. The body perceives a novel occurrence in the environment, and processes the information through higher brain centers, consciously choosing a behavioral response. This pathway allows the body to create a novel reaction to a new situation, but is slower than the top-down "auto-pilot" pathways. In a situation of real threat, this pathway could expose greater risk.

cover both ways of thinking about the placebo response, and avoid the negative connotations at the same time. Therefore, I have chosen to stick with "placebo response."

Before we move on to conditioning, I'd like to make one last point regarding expectancy.

Expectancy Plus

The expectancy theory has seemed such a strong predictor of placebo reactions that scientists may have overlooked some other factors that make important contributions. Donald Price and Howard Fields, focusing their attention on placebo pain relief, propose that desire may be as important a factor as expectancy. Placebo pain relief in clinical settings, with real patients, is often much more striking than placebo pain relief in psychology laboratory settings. One could propose that subjects in a lab experiment know that the pain will be temporary, while sick persons may have a much stronger motivation to be relieved of their pain. Price and Fields also looked at the handful of experiments where desire and expectancy were looked at separately, and at least one of those experiments showed that desire played as important a role as expectancy. (In chapter 12 I will go back to desire to get better as a major issue in the working of your inner pharmacy.)

In closing, I'd like to reiterate that expectancy theory gives us a very valuable, practical handle on the inner pharmacy. There are many different ways we can work with and alter people's expectancies. These all become potentially valuable tools for healing. At this point, it would seem that there is hardly any need for more theories. But, as we'll see in the next chapter, *conditioning theory* has also been highly successful in explaining and predicting certain aspects of the placebo response. So let's look at conditioning theory, too, and finally lay expectancy and conditioning side by side for comparison.

SIX

Conditioning Theory and the Placebo Response

"[Richard C.] Cabot's remark . . . that babes are not born with the desire to take a drug for every symptom, is quite wrong. The babe needs very much oral satisfaction for his symptoms, and the eternal babe within us, that comes to the forefront in illness often needs satisfaction by mouth. Such longings need to be considered in scientific treatment, too, or else the scientific view would be incomplete."

—Dr. M. B. Clyne, 1953

In this chapter we'll be studying significant scientific work which ties the placebo response to what psychologists call the *conditioned response.* This line of investigation is important, because it shows us what the *time sequence* of meaningful events in a person's life might have to do with the placebo response. Finally, we'll return to expectancy theory and see how it relates to contemporary and classical conditioning theory.

Classical Conditioning Theory

As you probably know from your school days, the father of psychological conditioning theory was the Russian scientist Ivan Pavlov (1849–1936). Aware that dogs routinely salivate when they are about to be fed, Pavlov experimented with a group of them by ringing a bell every time he gave them food. He discovered that after a while, the dogs would salivate when the bell rang, even if there was no food present.

We can use this simple example as a basis for understanding some key concepts of conditioning. At first, the salivation was what is called an *unconditioned response*: a normal bodily response to a particular stimulus (food). No training or special conditions are required for the body to perform an unconditioned response.

By contrast, the dogs' salivating in response only to the bell was a *conditioned response*: not natural or predictable at all. For this to happen, the dogs' bodies needed to undergo a series of changes. In particular, there had to be a linkage established between the *unconditioned stimulus* (the food) and the *conditioned stimulus* (the bell). One or two connections would not do the trick; the dogs had to be exposed to the food and the bell together dozens, maybe even hundreds, of times before the conditioning occurred. Such a series of events, which link the two stimuli together in the mind of the experimental animal and eventually results in conditioning, is called a *reinforcement schedule.*

So what happens if scientists continue ringing the bell for the dogs, but never give them food simultaneously? At first, the dogs, true to their conditioning experience, will go on salivating, but after a while, they will stop, having lost the association between the food and the bell. Scientists term this reversal of a reinforcement schedule *extinction.*

If we only study such examples from classical conditioning as Pavlov and his dogs, we might assume that it does not tell us anything about the placebo response—unless we find the response operating in dogs or rats. We have already learned that the symbolic significance of an event has a great deal to do with whether or not a placebo response will occur, and that symbolic significance, whatever it might involve, appears to require the brain's conscious processes. By contrast, we are not at all aware of the events that lead to classical conditioning; they occur at a totally subconscious level, and do not at all demand human consciousness.

Scientists today work with a substantially expanded model of conditioning, capable of taking into account both conscious and subconscious processes. If we employ this expanded model, many conscious processes could be viewed as types of conditioning—depending mainly on whether or not they can be meaningfully understood by looking at schedules of *reinforcement* or *extinction*.

Contemporary Conditioning Theory

Imagine that you're studying for a final exam, and you struggle for a week memorizing certain key points that are likely to be on the test. Now let's say that two months later, long after the course is over, someone asks you to name those key points; it's quite likely you'll have only imperfect recall, even though you passed the exam with flying colors. Applying conditioning theory to this episode, we see that studying hard for the test was a form of reinforcement schedule for memorizing the material. Then, when you stopped studying and turned your mind to other things, you went through an extinction phase. So conditioning theory would predict exactly what happened—first, your ability to pass the test; and second, your forgetting the information later on. But in this case the conditioning process involved the conscious mind—for surely no dog could have taken the test.

In fact, as long ago as the 1950s and 1960s, some scientists theorized that placebo effects might be due in some way to conditioning, but until the 1980s there were few facts to back up the idea.

Ader's Experiments

The major experiments that stimulated renewed interest in conditioning as a possible explanation of the placebo response were done in the 1980s by Dr. Robert Ader and his colleagues at the University of Rochester.

The first experiment was carried out in rats, with a drug called cyclophosphamide, which is normally used in cancer chemotherapy. It's an intensely powerful drug which basically knocks out the immune system for several days—a disadvantage because the animal treated with cyclophosphamide cannot fight off infection. Cyclophosphamide could be advantageous in treating such human diseases as rheumatoid arthritis and systemic lupus, which damage the body by an immune system gone out of control.

Dr. Ader administered cyclophosphamide to the rats, then measured their immune cells, finding, as predicted, that they dropped close to zero. He then began giving the rats cyclophosphamide and the artificial sweetener saccharin at the same time, combining the saccharin and cyclophosphamide exposures according to a variety of schedules. He also took into account that, when the rats were given saccharin alone, it did nothing at all to the immune system. Dr. Ader then tried the saccharin by itself and measured immune cell levels. The effect of saccharin on typical lab rats would lead us to predict there would be no change in the immune system. That is not what happened. Instead, saccharin acted very much like Pavlov's bell: It had become a conditioned stimulus as a result of being closely paired in the rats' experience with the unconditioned stimulus (cyclophosphamide). This meant that the conditioned rats given saccharin showed a drop in the number of immune cells. The drop was not down to zero, as happened with cyclophosphamide, but in some groups of rats it was substantial.

Dr. Ader discovered something even more important from the point of view of scientific theory: The drop-off in immune function with saccharin was not the same in the various groups of rats; it differed according to the schedule of reinforcement. In general, the more closely linked the cyclophasphamide had been with the saccharin, the greater the drop in immune cells; if there was a lesser connection, then there was not so dramatic a change in the immune cell count.

Basically, the experimental system worked exactly as it should have worked, if conditioning theory was a valid theory of what was happening. This encouraged Dr. Ader to try other experiments, examining how the connection between an active drug and a dummy drug could be strengthened over time (reinforcement) and also how long it took for the connection to disappear once the two were unlinked (extinction).

At that point, Ader's work had only involved laboratory animals. In one instance, he was able to try out a human application for his theory. You'll recall the case of Ruth, the girl with lupus, who responded so well to the cod liver oil and rose perfume in chapter 1. If only in that one case, the same principles that seemed to work in the laboratory with rats applied equally well to the human subject. Drs. Karen Olness and Ader carefully warn that it's dangerous to conclude too much from Ruth's case. Without a control patient, we have no way of knowing that she didn't simply need a lower dose of cyclophosphamide than average. A more recent study adds support to conditioning theory in human health:

The Vanilla Cure

Venezuelan physician Dr. Marianella Castes and her associates performed an experiment on forty-two children with asthma during a fifteen-day period. The conditioning group received two daily doses of a typical asthma medication in the form of a metered-dose inhaler, plus a vanilla aroma added as the conditioned stimulus. Another group of children were given the vanilla aroma and the medication, separately, at different times of the day, so that no conditioning would occur.

After fifteen days, when given vanilla aroma without any medication, the children in the conditioning group had measurable improvements in their lung functions. On average, this group displayed about a third the amount of improvement as the children with the "active" medication.

Dr. Castes's team made a very important observation during their research. Preliminary indications suggested that it was not the vanilla alone which functioned as a conditioned stimulus, since there was some evidence that the metered-dose inhaler device itself became associated with the medicine's effects in the minds of the children. That is, if the children used the same device, but it was filled with water instead of medicine, the spray by itself might be sufficient to produce some improvement in lung function. In this case, the level of improvement would again be about a third that of the "real" medicine. We can easily imagine how a person with chronic asthma, using his inhaler day in and day out, could become conditioned. This observation brings conditioning theory down to earth by showing that no special laboratory or experimental setting is needed to produce conditioning.

Placebo Response as Conditioning

Remember a common childhood event: The child hurts a finger, cries, and immediately demands a Band-Aid. What is going on here? According to conditioning theory, the child has in the past often had a pair of experiences. The child, let us say, had a cut which bled, Mother put on a Band-Aid, the cut stopped hurting. The unconditioned stimulus, the relief of pain, simply happened as a result of the natural healing powers of the body. But in the child's experience, it became linked with the conditioned stimulus: the Band-Aid. The child is now conditioned to experience pain relief if a Band-Aid is put on some body part that hurts. This could be the first experience that most of us, growing up, had with the placebo response!

The conditioned response may be even more general than this, and indeed probably is. This is the more general sequence:

1. Something starts to hurt.
2. Mother shows love and concern.
3. The hurting stops.

The child—and the adult, later on in life—has become powerfully conditioned to experience relief of pain or other unpleasant symptoms, whenever somebody expresses care and concern in a way that triggers an unconscious association with how Mother responded when the person was a small child.

Now, let's take the story one step further. Over many years, another association forms in the growing child's mind. When more serious illnesses or injuries happen, parents and doctors give the child medicine. In the vast majority of instances, the symptoms of the illness eventually disappear. Sometimes, this happens as cause and effect: The medicine makes the illness get better. Sometimes, as with the Band-Aid, it's simply natural healing powers at work, with the medicine simply along for the ride. To the conditioning response, what matters is the developing association linking the unconditioned stimulus (the relief of painful or scary symptoms) with the conditioned stimulus (medicine). The end result, according to conditioning theory, is an adult who will have a fair chance of getting better if given any medicine for a typical illness, even if the medicine is only a sugar pill.

Now let's suppose that at some point in life I had a serious disease that required a series of frequent, painful injections, and from which I later recovered. As a result, I came to believe injections were more powerful medicine than pills and that injections that were really painful were more powerful medicine than relatively painless ones. These types of associations have been shown in a variety of experiments to predict the intensity and frequency of placebo responses. For instance, savvy doctors and nurses wishing to give a strong placebo have, for many years, favored an injection of sterile water instead of a sterile salt solution because an injection of plain water stings more.

Modern conditioning theory is relatively indifferent to the question of whether previous experience is perceived by an animal at a conscious or an unconscious level. All that matters is that there is a sufficiently strong association, repeated enough times, and that nothing has occurred subsequently to extinguish the association. We may make the association subconsciously or consciously, as a matter of learned experience. A case in point is Albert, from the introduction, who insisted on antibiotics for a common cold, and, upon taking them, rapidly improved—despite the fact that colds are viral, and antibiotics do not kill viruses. It's probable that, by luck, Albert happened to twist the physician's arm precisely at that point when the cold had gotten as bad as it was going to get. No matter; antibiotics will in the future be powerful placebos for Albert, as a result of the conditioning (or learning) that has occurred.

In summarizing his views on the placebo effect as a conditioned response in 1997, Dr. Robert Ader gave further examples of studies by other investigators which seemed to confirm this theory:

- When patients with pain were switched from an analgesic drug to placebo, they remained pain-free long after the "die-away" period of the active drug.
- When given as the first medication administered in a study, aspirin and an anti-inflammatory drug called indomethacin were more effective than placebo; but they were no more effective when added as the second or third medication after placebo had already been given. Therefore, the history of prior exposures to drugs, both "active" and "inactive," was important in determining how the subject would react.
- Another study confirmed this point: The placebo was more effective when it followed active and effective drug therapy; active drugs were less effective when they followed ineffective treatment.
- Schizophrenics taken off their medications relapse more quickly than those taken off active medications but placed on placebo instead. Similarly, hypertensive people on a beta-blocker displayed normal blood pressure much longer when the beta-blocker was discontinued if they received a placebo than if they got no medicine at all. Again, the blood pressure response was much longer than the "wash-out" period it would have taken the "active" drug to leave the system.

Now, let's add expectancy to the equation.

Expectation or Conditioning: Which Is Valid?

We saw earlier that a good deal of placebo research fits with an expectancy theory. There is an obvious problem in trying to decide whether experimental data suggest that a conditioning theory is more plausible than expectation theory or vice versa. In most instances, the same factors that create a conditioning reinforcement schedule will also create conscious expectations in the minds of human subjects. We have to assume that Dr. Ader's rats did not *expect* to have a drop in the number of their immune cells when they took saccharin following the reinforcement schedule with the saccharin/cyclophosphamide pairing. In that regard they were different from the subjects of most experiments involving placebos in humans.

In recent years, a few researchers have tried to design experiments that could put conditioning and expectation to the test and declare a clear winner. To create the ideal test situation, the experiments had to be done in the psychology laboratory. That leads to a warning we must keep in mind. The vast bulk of modern placebo research shows that the situation or setting in which we find ourselves is a more potent predictor of any placebo response than most long-standing personality traits. The more important the setting, the harder it is to create in a laboratory an experimental situation that appropriately mimics what happens to real patients suffering from real illnesses.

It's common to do studies of the placebo response in a psychology laboratory, where pain is artificially induced by an electric shock or by applying a tourniquet to one arm. Subjects of these experiments know that they are in an artificial setting, that they have no disease, and that once the experiment is over, the pain will be gone. How well could we apply findings from an experiment like this to patients who suffer from real diseases, and who cannot know whether or not their pain or other symptoms will be cured in the future? The psychology of the two situations is so different that knowing how the inner pharmacy works in one setting may provide us with very few clues of how it would work in the other.

Still, so long as we bear this warning in mind, we have the potential advantage that laboratory experiments can be designed with a care, precision, and predictability that we could simply never attain in the real world of illness and symptoms. And some of these laboratory experiments have been so cleverly conducted that they are worth our time.

A Pain in the Arm

A group in Victoria, Australia, led by Dr. Nicholas Voudouris, began a series of studies by creating a fascinating experimental model. The scientists told their subjects that they wanted to test the properties of a new analgesic cream, which in all cases was actually a placebo. They created pain on the skin of the arm by applying an electric current (thereby allowing precise measurement of the intensity of the pain stimulus) and also very carefully standardized the amount of current given to reproduce exactly a specific level of subjective pain.

The experiment was done with each subject serving as his or her own control, so that it was literally a *two-armed* study. The subjects had cream applied to one arm only, and the electric-current pad was placed on both. They were supposed to report whether the pain they had in one arm was different from the pain in the other.

Dr. Voudouris and his team wanted to test expectancy theory against conditioning theory, so they needed to expose some of their subjects to an "expectancy situation" and others to a "conditioning situation." They reasoned that what they told the subjects about the cream before the experiment could serve as a verbal expectancy condition—so they gave some subjects a written consent form which described the cream as a potent analgesic which would kill pain, while others received a written form stating that they would be in a control group and would be getting a neutral cream which had no effect on pain. They next reasoned that when the subjects received the cream, the conditioning situation would arise based on their prior experience with pain relief. Some of the subjects, while told that they were getting the same current in both arms, actually got substantially less current in the arm with the cream, creating the impression that the cream was reducing the pain. Then, they underwent a measurement session in which the current was kept at higher levels to see if the conditioned subjects reported less pain or the same pain in the arm with the cream after previously being exposed to the conditioning.

The scientists ended up with four categories of subjects: expectancy only; conditioning only; both expectancy and conditioning; and neither.

Their results came out strongly in favor of conditioning. Both of the conditioning groups reported less pain in the arm that had the cream, compared to the other arm. Adding the expectancy to the conditioning did not do more to reduce pain than did conditioning alone. Expectancy alone did nothing to reduce pain.

Dr. Voudouris and his group frankly acknowledged the potential limits of this study. They noted that one could not make so clear a distinction between conditioning and expectancy. The actual experience with the pain apparently getting less in the arm with the cream, besides creating a conditioning situation, also changed the expectancy of the subjects. One could imagine that this actual experience was more powerful in forming expectancy than whatever words were written on a form that had been given some time ago. Therefore, to be completely accurate, the Voudouris study did not so much show that conditioning worked better than expectancy, as it showed that the actual experience created a more powerful placebo response than written words.

Aware of this problem, Guy Montgomery and Dr. Irving Kirsch at the University of Connecticut set out to replicate as closely as possible Dr. Voudouris's experiments with an added wrinkle: two different conditioning groups. In each case, the current was turned down lower when the placebo cream was applied. But one group was kept in the dark about this, while the other group was told it would happen.

The two researchers reasoned that if the placebo effect worked in the same way that Pavlov's dogs learned to salivate when the bell rang, all that mattered was the constant pairing of the cream with the lessening of pain—meaning that what the subjects consciously thought could not matter. On the other hand, if what matters is expectancy, then telling the subjects that the current was being turned down would produce a vastly different expectancy.

Montgomery and Kirsch also added an extinction group. They continued to give this group the full level of electric current, even after applying the placebo cream. By Pavlovian reasoning, when the placebo stimulus was constantly paired with the failure to achieve pain relief, extinction rather than reinforcement would occur and the placebo effect would gradually disappear. But Montgomery and Kirsch realized that if the placebo effect works as we think it does, it ought to be self-reinforcing. If I take a placebo pill, and afterward feel better, then, when I take a placebo pill in the future, I will expect to feel better again. Thus, if a positive placebo response takes place and leads the subject to expect a positive response, then the placebo effect ought to resist Pavlovian extinction.

Finally, since they were interested in comparing expectancy to conditioning, Montgomery and Kirsch asked all their subjects just how much pain they expected to feel with and without the placebo cream. The results of this complicated set of experiments strongly supported an expectancy model. Telling the subjects that the current would be turned down led to much less placebo response than not telling them. The extinction trial series actually led to an increase, and not a disappearance, of the placebo effect. When Montgomery and Kirsch looked at the stated expectations of all the subjects, they found that they correlated almost exactly with the placebo responses. Therefore, expectancy accounted for all the observations, leading to the conclusions that if conditioning has any role at all, it works by creating an expectancy that one will feel better after taking a placebo.

Scheduling: The Relationship Between Expectancy and Conditioning

I do not believe that any one set of experiments is the last word on expectancy and conditioning as theories of the placebo response. The best perspective on the subject today is that each has something important to teach us. (We should keep in mind Fisher and Greenberg's warning that the placebo response may well be the single most complex behavioral phenomenon ever studied by psychologists and medical scientists; so we should not be surprised if any one theory turns out to be incomplete.)

Conditioning requires that we look not only at what we give the patient today, but also at the patient's past history. It also requires that we thoroughly examine the time schedules for treatments in the laboratory and the physician's office. For all we know, giving a medicine three times a day, or for three weeks, is a very powerful conditioning stimulus, while giving exactly the same medicine twice a day, or for two weeks, is not a sufficient reinforcement schedule for conditioning to occur.

The fact is that very few studies of the placebo response, or of active drugs for that matter, have carefully looked at these kinds of scheduling issues. Before now, when medical scientists considered the impact of how many times a medicine was taken each day, they usually had only one thing in mind: If we have to take our medicines three or four times a day, we tend to forget or to give up; while if we have to take them only once or twice a day, we are more likely to be "compliant." But what if it turns out that the more often we take the medicine, compliance goes down, yet the conditioned response goes up? Then we would have to study carefully the pros and cons of compliance and conditioning. For some people the fewer-times-a-day approach might be best; for others the more-times-per-day approach might be superior.

In many ways, it need not concern us much whether expectancy or conditioning theory is true. Remember the top-down vs. bottom-up model that was used to explain the expectancy theory? If you go back and look at that model carefully, you'll see that you only have to modify a couple of features and it could be used just as well for conditioning theory. (In expectancy theory, all we care about is that the top-down healing patterns are stored in the brain's memory files, while in conditioning theory we study how those patterns might get laid down in the files to begin with.) So the two theories may be describing the same process, but from two slightly different vantage points.

Though both expectancy theory and conditioning theory provide us with important clues, they do not address another key portion of the mystery of the placebo response: the idea of *symbolic significance* that we introduced in our definition back in chapter 1. What does all this *mean* to the person who is undergoing the response? I'll address this in the next chapter and, in the process, propose a new model for understanding the placebo response and the inner pharmacy.

SEVEN

The Meaning Model

"It is not enough for [the physician] to take an adequate history or make an adequate physical examination. We must also try to understand the inner needs and longings of our patients, or else all well-meant treatment with fine names, after high-sounding diagnoses, will be a placebo for the satisfaction of our own needs."

—Dr. M. B. Clyne, 1953

Conditioning theory does not require the healer to know anything about the person involved in an experiment; you simply have to be familiar with her past history of exposure to various stimuli. Expectancy theory requires you to be aware of a single factor of concern in the person's mind: what he expects to happen in the future. Neither theory asks a more profound question: What does the illness, and its treatment, mean to the person? In this chapter, starting with the anecdote below, we'll see why the meaning issue may be pivotal to unraveling the mystery of the inner pharmacy.

Dr. Henry Beecher and the Wounded Soldiers

You've already read about Dr. Henry Beecher, who, in 1955, published a breakthrough article entitled "The Powerful Placebo" in a major medical journal. It was perhaps the first article by a mainstream investigator to lend legitimacy to the placebo as worthy of scientific study.

What led Beecher to become interested in how placebos relieve pain? He explained that his experiences as a military physician in World War II first impressed on him the potential power of the mind over the body.

He observed seriously wounded infantrymen brought from the front to the field hospitals. He then calculated—based on his peacetime experiences—how severe the pain would be for a civilian who had suffered a similar degree of injury, say, in a traffic or industrial accident. Dr. Beecher was astounded to see that often these soldiers claimed to feel far less pain and complained less than civilians would have.

Dr. Beecher realized that, while the tissue damage to the soldier and the civilian might have been identical, the *meaning* of the pain in the two situations was totally different. Pain for the civilian was an unmitigated disaster; it meant an inability to go about one's daily occupation, plus the likelihood of having to submit to major surgery, followed by a prolonged convalescence—and in some cases was accompanied by the threat of loss of employment and financial ruin. To the soldiers, the pain was a much more hopeful event. It meant, first, that they had not been killed; and second, that they were at least temporarily relieved of the threat of death on the front lines. Dr. Beecher hypothesized that this different meaning attached to the pain affected not only how much his patients complained, but also how much pain they actually experienced. This led him to wonder what other mental influences that changed the meaning of the illness experience for the patient might have a measurable effect on pain level.

Symbolic Significance and the Meaning Model

The human mind-body system could be described as "an ignoring machine." At any given moment, thousands of processes take place inside our bodies. And at that same moment, almost an infinite number of things occur in the environment around us. Yet we ignore most of this information and are highly selective about what we attend to, whether we are conscious of it or not. This "tunnel vision" is ultimately a blessing. We could never make sense of the mass of information we would be required each second to digest from the environment and would probably go mad. That is why we select very carefully the things to which we assign symbolic meaning.

What have we learned from scientific studies that might help us better to understand what causes people to attach special significance to some symbols and not to others? One model especially useful in organizing the large body of available information is the *meaning model*, which goes as follows:

> **An encounter with a healer is most likely to produce a positive placebo response when it changes the meaning of the illness experience for that individual in a positive direction.**
>
> **The meaning of the illness experience most likely changes in a positive direction when these three things happen:**
>
> - **The individual is listened to and receives an explanation for the illness that makes sense.**
> - **The individual feels care and concern being expressed by the healer and others in the environment.**
> - **The individual feels an enhanced sense of mastery or control over the illness or its symptoms.**

But before we look more closely at the three elements of the meaning model, we should note other aspects of the model. First, because we are most interested in healing, we have stressed positive results. But of course, as we've seen in cases like Mrs. S.—who mistakenly thought a physician had announced she was going to die, and proceeded to do so—the placebo response could be *any change* in the patient's health status. Thus, if the patient leaves an encounter with a so-called healer feeling more bewildered than ever about the illness, uncared for, and helpless, then we would expect our old bugaboo the nocebo effect to occur just as readily.

I will talk more about negative placebo responses in the next chapter.

Right now, we should keep in mind that an unpleasant encounter with a physician can greatly affect a person's health.

The second point is that while the meaning model breaks down into the three elements, they are often closely intermingled. Let's look at a now-classic 1960s study by Dr. Lawrence Egbert and fellow anesthesiologists at Harvard Medical School.

The Placebo Response Without the Placebo

Dr. Egbert's team selected ninety-seven patients about to undergo major abdominal surgery for various conditions and divided them into two groups. The control group got the standard anesthesia presurgery visit, in which the anesthesiologist visits the patient, takes a succinct medical history, and does a brief physical exam. By contrast, the experimental group received an enhanced visit from the anesthesiologist in which the subject of pain after surgery was dealt with at some length.

The anesthesiologists sent this message to the experimental group: "You are, as I'm sure you know, going to have pain after surgery. I want to stress that the pain is normal and to be expected from a surgery like yours. There are a number of things you yourself can do to reduce the pain, such as turning in bed in a certain way or holding your sides when you cough. I'm going to give you a list of those things. Also, the doctors have ordered very strong pain medicine for you. Don't hesitate to ask for it when you need it. The nurses here are always very concerned and will respond very quickly if you let them know you need help with your pain."

The results of the experiment were striking. Egbert and his colleagues kept track of the amount of narcotic used by the two groups, and found that the experimental group used one-half as much pain medicine as the control group in total. The nurses did not know who was who, and so there could have been no bias in giving the medication. In addition, the surgeons, who weren't even aware the test was being conducted, discharged the experimental patients, on average, two days earlier than the control patients. Since the patients had very similar surgeries and had been randomly assigned to the two groups, Egbert argued that these differences were unlikely to be due to how much relative pain the patients experienced. Instead, his group asserted they had produced a "placebo effect without a placebo." Indeed, this study is a classic precisely because the Egbert group was among the first to realize the placebo response was conceptually independent from the use of dummy medicines.

Let's apply the meaning model to the Egbert study and see what might have happened. We have to admit that there could have been a pain relief effect that was separate from the placebo response. This would be a "clinic effect": a superior health outcome due not to symbolic significance, but rather because the patients were being closely watched and treated by skilled physicians. If the patients used the pain-reduction techniques described by the anesthesiologists, they might have had less pain for purely physical reasons and as a result needed less medication. The patients simply got more good advice and followed it.

Assuming there was at least some placebo component to explain the strikingly positive findings, we can see that the anesthesiologists combined all three elements of the meaning model. They talked about postoperative pain, which surgeons back in the 1960s often did not. It was commonplace to dismiss the pain as "you'll feel a little sore."

After the anesthesiologist's visit, the patient could deal with the pain openly, and need no longer fear it as something so terrible that it did not even have a name (meaningful explanation). The physicians then expressed compassion by their obvious desire to help and by the extra time they spent with the patients (care and concern). They emphasized that they were not the only caring persons around and that the nurses could also be relied on. And, finally, by stressing what the patients could do for themselves, they left their patients much less helpless and more in control (mastery and control). The patients were also buoyed by the awareness that aid was available if their own sense of control flagged.

If we were to ask which specific way of creating a positive meaning was at work in the Egbert experiment, we would have to answer that we don't know. Did the explanations work because they were good explanations, or because they made the patient feel more cared for, or because they enhanced the patients' sense of control? In one sense, the experimental design was insufficient, because it does not allow us to make these fine distinctions. In another sense, it was excellent, because now we have a proven program that physicians and nurses can use to reduce postoperative pain. In the real world of medical treatment, explanations, care and concern, and mastery and control all go hand-in-hand. So the advantage of the meaning model is that we can weave the three elements together for treatment effectiveness, or else we can separate them for designing better research in the future.

Explanation and the Importance of Stories

Tongue partly in cheek, I have called the human mind-body unit an ignoring machine. More importantly, it's a meaning-making machine. As I've said, we humans are animals who go around the world striving to construct meaning out of our experiences, to make some sense of whatever happens to us. How well we feel, how well we function—and ultimately how successful we deem our lives to have been—are all tied up with the meaning we attach to our experiences and our lives.

A prominent psychologist, Jerome Bruner, has concluded that the major way we make meaning of our lives is to tell stories. Stories have a beginning and an ending; they have structure; things happen that cause other things to happen in a way suggesting we can predict and control certain events.

We are so used to thinking in stories, we can easily forget that the raw data with which the world presents us often lack clear beginnings, endings, causes, and effects. Those are generally things we construct with our minds and our stories, not things that the world hands to us on a platter. We construct our image of the world in a way that attaches meaning to things in our lives.

We've learned that most scientists assume knowledge of the world comes only from scientific experiment and research—that stories are anecdotal and hence never give us any real knowledge. By contrast, Bruner suggests that stories are the most basic, fundamental, and universal way humans have of making sense of the world. Bruner further states that science is itself just a unique and disciplined way of storytelling.

Quite recently, medical investigators have become deeply interested in the stories that sick persons construct about their illnesses and healing. The results of this line of research are somewhat promising even though the research remains in its infancy. For instance, physician Eric Cassell and sociologist Arthur Frank both have argued that we commonly make a mistake in confusing the ideas of pain and suffering. Two people could have equal amounts of pain, but one may be suffering only slightly while the other may be suffering terribly. The difference is the story that each person constructs around the pain.

A story of suffering is a story of meaninglessness, isolation, and hopelessness. Suffering may persist even though the patient gets extensive medical treatment, so long as the story does not change. The suffering may lighten considerably if the patient can find a way to tell a different story. Telling your story and being listened to and understood may well be a crucial aspect of healing.

Chapter 1 discussed another body of medical research that may have to do with the explanations that patients construct, or receive, for their illnesses. Several different studies demonstrated that whether patients got better after seeing the physician depended on how well the patients felt the physicians listened to them during the original visit.

These "being listened to" studies seem to fall under the heading of care and concern, not explanation. If I listen to you and spend more time to hear your story in detail, I am simply showing that I care about you. Yet I suggest that these findings cross over into the explanation category as well.

If a physician offers me an explanation for my illness, what makes it a *satisfactory* explanation? It seems reasonable that if he has carefully listened to me, I will have a much higher level of confidence that he is explaining *my* illness, and is not simply handing me a stock explanation off the shelf. If I have a sympathetic and careful listener, I will also go into more detail in my story. In telling it I may do a better job of explaining to myself (as well as to the physician) what is the matter with me. When real listening has occurred, the improved explanation is a joint product of the physician's and the patient's efforts.

Care and Concern

Care and compassion can be delivered in several ways. The healer may be the one expressing care and concern. She may be surrounded by a group of others who reinforce that compassion. (There are many emotionally distant physicians who have probably managed to trigger positive placebo responses by hiring very warm and caring nurses and receptionists.) Finally, the sick person's family and friends may be helped to show more care and concern as a result of the healing encounter. In some American Indian and African tribal cultures, a healing ceremony will often be an occasion for an entire village to gather around the sick person to demonstrate tangible support and caring.

What evidence have we to show that care and concern can exert a healing influence? The data are quite sketchy. Perhaps the most striking studies are those of the role of the doula in childbirth. A doula is a labor companion who has no specific health skills or training, but whose role is simply to be with the woman who is having the baby.

"I Don't Want to Be Alone"

American pediatricians Marshall Klaus and John Kennell first became interested in the effect of the doula after looking at birth practices in a large Central American hospital. They noted that in the native culture, women were usually kept company constantly throughout the labor process. But in the name of sterility and efficiency, the new hospital ended up herding most laboring women into small rooms, where they were alone and were checked by nurses only at intervals.

Drs. Klaus and Kennell and their colleagues decided to train some women as doulas and to assign these doulas randomly to half the patients. Despite the fact that the doulas had been taught no medical or nursing skills, and had never met the women prior to labor, the study found notable differences in the two groups. The doula patients had shorter and easier labors, and both the mothers and the infants had fewer complications after birth. The team of pediatricians later found a U.S. hospital where women labored alone and produced equally impressive results when the doulas were introduced there.

Why should the doula make a difference? The best answer we can provide comes from a personal anecdote.

The Surprise Visitor

A pediatrician friend—whom we'll call Dr. Shaw—was told that she needed to have surgery. She was admitted to the hospital where she did much of her work, and was given a private room.

As she lay in bed the night before surgery, Dr. Shaw realized she was terrified. She knew she shouldn't have been. She was a physician and knew all about the surgery and the lack of any serious or unusual risk involved. But she was terrified anyway.

Suddenly there was a knock at the door, which opened to reveal a woman named Dr. Sharma, who had come from her native India to train as a specialist in pediatric heart disease. Dr. Shaw was amazed to see that Dr. Sharma was carrying a sleeping bag and a robe. "What are you doing here?" Dr. Shaw demanded, her astonishment getting the better of her manners.

"I am going to sleep in your room tonight," replied Dr. Sharma. "In India we would never let a person sleep alone on the night before surgery. Don't worry, I won't disturb you or make any noise; I'll just sleep here in the corner."

"At that moment," Dr. Shaw reported later, "I felt a totally unexpected and yet massively powerful calm come over me. I had not even realized how much tension had crept into my body until I suddenly felt it all draining away in an instant—simply because another caring human being was with me."

Another interesting tidbit of research helps explain how care and compassion might be related to healing. I mention it with some hesitancy because it's research that was done in the psychology laboratory, with the limitations that artificial situations impose. This research should be viewed as preliminary and should be confirmed in illness situations. Still, it is so intriguing that it should be mentioned.

The Mother Teresa Experiment

Psychologist David McClelland of Harvard University was the head of a team studying the relationship between environmental signals and a particular germ-fighting antibody, a protein called immunoglobulin A, produced by the salivary gland in the mouth (salivary IgA or "SIgA" for short). Since many disease-causing germs first enter through the mouth, SIgA could be seen as one of the body's first lines of defense against such minor illnesses as the common cold. SIgA was useful for McClelland's research because it is easy to measure. All a subject has to do is spit into a test tube to get a sample for analysis.

McClelland's group devised an experiment. A group of student volunteers' SIgA levels were measured before and after they watched a videotape of Mother Teresa aiding the impoverished ill in Calcutta. After the tape concluded, students' reactions to it were found to range across the board. Some disliked it. Some said it made them extremely depressed. Others claimed the film disgusted them with its vivid portrayal of the filth and squalor of the Calcutta slums. But all agreed that the predominant qualities depicted in the film were care and compassion. All students, even those who didn't like it, showed a significant rise in their levels of SIgA after the movie.

Immediately after the screening, McClelland divided the students randomly into two groups. The experimental group was asked to perform a one-hour task, designed to reinforce and prolong the message of caring. The students were requested to write an essay about a personal event earlier in their lives that seemed to display the same sort of compassion shown in the film. The control group was given a distracting task, doing math problems, for example. When another hour had passed, their SIgA was measured again.

After this second phase of the experiment, the two groups showed marked differences. Both groups had at first shown a rise in SIgA after seeing the movie. For the control group, this rise had disappeared one hour later. They were back to their previous baseline level. But the reinforced group continued to show a higher level of SIgA even after the additional hour had elapsed.

If we bear in mind all the warnings about applying the study to medical settings without further proof, the McClelland research still suggests how care and concern might be translated into health improvement. First, it raises the possibility that exposure to a caring environment might stimulate the secretion of healing or health-preserving substances by the body's inner pharmacy. Second, it shows that reinforcing messages can again trigger high levels of these substances later on.

Imagine that a patient feels cared for by a physician or a medical team and then is told to take a pill every day for two weeks. It would not be surprising if the pill was to serve as a tangible reminder of the care and compassion shown by the physician, and of the positive healing relationship that had been established. After all, one of Park and Covi's subjects did report in chapter 3 that each time she took her placebo pills, she was reminded positively of how she was helping herself.

Taking the pill could be a *reinforcing task* which helps to keep the SIgA levels high for the entire two weeks, which is totally in keeping with the conditioning theories we discussed in chapter 6. Whether it actually happens in medical settings remains to be shown, but it would seem important to do these studies to find out.

Mastery and Control

Control and mastery can happen in two ways. First, the patient might feel that she has personal control over the illness. Second, she could decide that even though she personally has almost no control, some other powerful persons whom she trusts do.

This second mechanism may have been operating in a classic study of heart attack victims in Israel. The patients who did well were able to release control and trust either in their physicians or their religious faith. Here we will focus principally on evidence that enhanced personal control over symptoms can promote healing.

Mastery as Healer

Perhaps the most important facts on mastery as healing come from a series of studies conducted by Drs. Sheldon Greenfield and Sherrie Kaplan and their colleagues. They began studying patients who suffered from stomach and bowel disorders, but later discovered virtually the same things happened when they looked at patients with other chronic diseases in various parts of the country.

Greenfield and Kaplan divided these first subjects randomly into two groups. The mastery group was given a special training session. The goal of the session was to help these patients learn to take an active role in their clinic visits by asking more questions, being more directive with their physicians, and achieving great clarity about what they wanted.

The study team went over the chart records of the last several visits to identify things the patients wanted to talk about. Did they know why they were taking the medicines that had been prescribed? Were there any side effects of the medicines they had been hesitant to mention? Did they want more information about nutrition? Then the patients were led through a practice session to get them ready to be more assertive in their next visit with the doctor.

The control group also had a session with the study team, taking the same amount of time. The focus here was not at all on mastery. These patients were instead given educational sessions about their diseases. No review of their charts and no practice sessions occurred.

The study team had already videotaped clinic visits with all of the patients; they also videotaped the following clinic visit. The videotapes showed that the patients in the mastery group had in fact learned their lessons. Compared both to their earlier visit and also to the control group, they asked more questions and generally took more charge of the discussion.

The change in the mastery group of patients was not confined to the clinic visit. In the month following the training session, the group reported that they had had much less interference of their bowel symptoms in their daily lives and activities. Their symptoms didn't go away, but they were much less of a hindrance.

On the other hand, the control group did learn more about their illness, and when compared with the mastery group, clearly had better basic knowledge. During the next month, that didn't translate into an improvement in their health or functioning.

Greenfield and Kaplan wondered if the difference could have come from differences in satisfaction. Perhaps, the mastery patients were more satisfied with their clinic visits. Was it possible that greater satisfaction, and not mastery, had exerted the healing influence? As it turned out, both mastery and control groups expressed equal levels of satisfaction with their clinic visits and with the training sessions. The one difference was that the mastery group, having seen what it was like to be more in control, expressed a preference in the future for proactive clinic visits and indicated no desire to return to the more passive mode. The satisfaction scores of the physicians were not the same: Some of the physicians expressed a definite dissatisfaction for the more assertive patients, who presumably demanded more of their time and energy.

Greenfield, Kaplan, and their colleagues went on to test hypertensive and diabetic patients. A summary of their findings revealed that instructing patients to be more in control of their medical care produced better functional health results. Those patients lost fewer days from work, had fewer limits imposed by their illness on their normal activities, and reported that they simply *felt* healthier overall. At the same time, such measurements of their bodily functions as blood pressure for the hypertensives and blood sugar for the diabetics improved more in the group with the greater-control training program.

How Does Meaning Heal?

When, as a result of being in a healing environment, the *meaning* of the illness experience becomes more positive, then a positive placebo response is more likely to happen. And we have seen that the more positive meaning could consist of one of or any combination of three factors: meaningful explanation; care and concern; or mastery and control.

We have also seen one hint of what might be happening chemically in the patient's body to translate these changes in meaning into processes that are known to affect health outcomes: the increase in SIgA in the McClelland study. For the most part we have not investigated the biochemical processes that might solve the puzzle of how changed meaning stimulates the inner pharmacy. We will explore that question in a later chapter. First, we need to return to the flip side of the placebo coin: the nocebo.

EIGHT

The Nocebo Effect

"A lady, a patient, informed me that opium administered in any way, caused great restlessness, violent headache, and vomiting. Having of necessity to use it in her case, I prescribed it under the usual medical name, Tincture Opii. The following day I found that her account of its effects were correct, as she had passed a very restless night, with violent headache and vomiting. From her husband, I learned that she was in the habit of reading and commenting upon all the prescriptions of the different physicians who had previously attended her. After a few days I had recourse to the same remedy under a new name (Tincture Thebacia). Now, under this new term, I gave her opium for a length of time without producing the smallest inordinate action, and without the least symptoms of headache or vomiting, but on the contrary, she slept soundly and improved in health. She also spoke in the highest terms of this new remedy . . . "

—Dr. John C. Gunn, 1861

By now you're familiar with the nocebo effect (from the Latin "I shall harm"):

A situation in which a negative expectation leads to a greater likelihood that ill health will result.

As Dr. Gunn appreciated many years ago, his patient's expectation that some substance called "Tincture Opii" would cause her to feel sick was enough to produce the actual symptoms—and that the reaction had nothing to do with the actual chemical composition of the substance, as calling the same chemical by a different name made the symptoms disappear. Just what is the nocebo effect?

Patty's Big Scare

One cold winter morning Patty, a thirty-seven-year-old mother of three, woke with vaginal bleeding. This was peculiar because her period had ended ten days before, and she considered herself very regular. In fact, she often joked with her friends that the only certain things in life were death, taxes, and the exact dates of her periods. Two days later, with the bleeding having gotten even heavier, she called her gynecologist, Dr. Paluzzi.

Patty had a great relationship with the warm, intelligent, and affable physician. It was reaching Dr. Paluzzi that was the problem. The size of her practice often made it difficult to talk directly to her. Sheila Garrison, one of the office nurses, acted as the gatekeeper for all incoming calls and (seemed to) enjoy this position of power. Sheila began by matter-of-factly asking Patty a series of questions: Are you dizzy or short of breath? nauseated? sweats or chills? Patty was unsettled by Sheila's nonchalance. After five minutes, she asked the nurse for a more definite sense of the problem: "Can you tell me anything about what you think it could be?"

"Oh, let's see. It could be something as simple as an irregular cycle or as serious as cancer."

Cancer? The word nearly knocked the wind out of Patty. When she was in her early twenties and just out of college, she'd had surgery for endometriosis. The procedure was successful, but she'd been told that it left her at greater risk for sterility and cancer, with the risks increasing as she got older. Feeling weak and helpless, Patty hung up the phone. Negative thoughts kept creeping into her head. *It's probably nothing, just an irregular cycle, but what if it's bad news? My God, what if it is cancer? How will Paul and the kids take it? How will I handle it?* The more she thought about the conversation with Sheila, the more upset she became.

Two hours later, Patty still hadn't received a call back from Dr. Paluzzi's office, so she decided to try her other physician, Dr. Graubert, an internist who integrated elements of holistic medicine into his practice. Fortunately, Dr. Graubert came on the line right away, providing Patty with an almost immediate sense of relief. He asked pertinent questions and listened patiently to her answers.

"Hmmm . . . at your age you're certainly not premenopausal," he told her thoughtfully. "But you'd be surprised how easily your body can be affected by different things: trauma, work, stress. Have you been stressed lately?"

"Well . . . "

With a little prompting from Dr. Graubert, Patty admitted to total exhaustion, raising three kids, always another load of laundry to do, dinner to cook, errands to run, and never feeling she had time for herself. And as supportive as her husband was, Paul didn't seem to know what to do to help her.

"It sounds like you need to relax," Dr. Graubert counseled her. "Now, don't misunderstand—if the situation gets worse over the next few days, I definitely want you to go see Dr. Paluzzi. But do me a favor first. Take a little time off on your own today. Go for a hike in the mountains. Get your mind off things. And when this thing passes over, I want you to set up an appointment so that we can talk some more, okay?"

"Okay, thanks so much for taking the time to talk to me, Dr. Graubert."

She hung up the phone and let out a deep sigh. The conversation was exactly what she needed: the reassuring voice of someone she trusted telling her things would be okay. Patty did go for a long walk that day, and when she woke up the next morning, the bleeding had stopped. Was it just coincidence? She knew her improvement might have resulted from any number of factors, but she liked to think it was because she had called a physician who cared and listened.

The Medical Hex

In one day, Patty had two very different experiences with medical environments. The second, with Dr. Graubert, was a good example of the meaning model in action. As a result of her phone call with Graubert, Patty felt listened to, cared about, and more in control of her stressful life. Based on our model, this change could account for her inner pharmacy's stopping the bleeding when it did. But suppose that Dr. Graubert had been off at the hospital on an emergency, and the only medical conversation Patty had that day was with the nurse, Sheila Garrison. Then what would have happened?

It seems probable that Patty would have been the victim of what Dr. Andrew Weil calls "medical hexing." Dr. Weil compares these almost always unintentional expressions of medical pessimism to true hexes in primitive cultures, where a person may actually sicken and die as a result of believing a curse has been placed upon him by a powerful sorcerer. Certainly, the sinking feeling that Patty experienced after she got off the phone with Sheila was probably similar to what sufferers of "voodoo death" endure immediately after being hexed.

Nocebo: What Is Its Link to the Placebo Response?

Dr. Robert Hahn, who has studied the nocebo effect extensively, emphasizes that it is important to distinguish a true nocebo effect from a placebo side effect. Consider Adrienne and Bernice.

Let's say Adrienne was one of the subjects in Dr. Luparello's asthma experiment, which we talked about in chapter 5. Adrienne was given medicine that helps asthmatics breathe better, but she was told that it would make her breathing worse. As a result, she began wheezing and coughing. By contrast, Bernice, in another experiment involving a new antibiotic for bladder infections, was placed in the placebo group without her knowledge. While taking the placebo, Bernice got rid of her bladder symptoms, but she also became nauseated. Asked about this, she assumed that the new medicine had made her nauseated. After all, she knew it was a common side effect of drugs.

By Hahn's definition, Adrienne had a true nocebo effect. She expected to get worse and did, according to her expectation. Bernice, by contrast, expected to get better and indeed improved overall, but suffered side effects in the process. To Hahn, only a case like Adrienne's—which is the true opposite of the positive placebo response—would legitimately be called a nocebo effect.

Fortunately, Adrienne's nocebo response, as well as Patty's, was short-lived. Let's suppose now that they had been long-term.

Can the Nocebo Effect Kill?

We spoke of Dr. Andrew Weil's referring to the nocebo effect as "medical hexing," thereby relating it to the phenomenon of "voodoo death" in cultures with strong beliefs in the power of sorcerers. Presumably, on being told that a death hex had been cast upon them, some individuals from voodoo societies sickened and died, despite the absence of any disease or specific cause of death that Western medicine could detect. Today, the research on voodoo death, originally reported as scientific fact by the physiologist Walter Cannon in 1942, has come under fire. Anthropologists familiar with primitive cultures suggest that Western scientists were hoodwinked by romantic tales and that these deaths are actually mythical.

While voodoo death was believed to be real, American scientists studied the heart and discovered some mechanisms that could logically lead from severe emotional stress to a fatal irregularity in the heart's rhythm. And at least in one case, recorded by a careful observer in a setting where the patient was closely monitored, death seems to have arisen as a result of a nocebo effect. This is the case we've already seen, of Dr. Lown and Mrs. S. in chapter 1. Mrs. S's "death from abbreviation" appears to be a pure nocebo effect.

What are some other examples of nocebo effects? Dr. Hahn, among his studies of the medical literature, cites so-called instances of mass hysteria that occur regularly in factories, offices, and schools.

The Nocebo Effect and Medical Mass Hysteria

Incidents of medical mass hysteria happen fairly often and probably go unreported much of the time. A perfect example is the incident described below.

The East Templeton Toxin

On the morning of May 20, 1981, 102 East Templeton, Massachusetts, elementary school students boarded buses and were taken to a nearby regional high school, where they would rehearse their choral roles in an annual spring concert to be held at the school that evening. When they arrived, they joined three hundred students from other schools in the high school auditorium.

Suddenly, after half an hour of rehearsing, several students fell to the floor, grabbing their throats and abdomens and complaining of nausea, stomach pain, and difficulty breathing. Teachers escorted the stricken outside, but, when more and more students inside collapsed, the fire department was called. In the end, forty-one students developed symptoms similar to the first group but with the addition of dizziness, weakness, itchy eyes, and fainting. The students were brought to the hospital, checked out, and declared well enough to perform at the concert. Interestingly, all but one of those affected were from East Templeton. The drama didn't end there.

During the evening performance, a girl in the first row of the chorus collapsed, setting off a second chain reaction similar to the events of the morning, although this time there were also complaints of paralysis of the limbs. A total of twenty-nine students developed symptoms during the evening performance. They were rushed back to the hospital—yet emergency room physicians reported they all had normal physical exams, X-rays, and lab tests. Even so, fifteen of the most severely afflicted children were kept overnight in a hospital due to persistent nausea.

Two days later, a follow-up report from the emergency room stated that urine samples taken from thirteen of the children contained a trace amount of a chemical (n-butylbenzine sulfonamide) found in both insecticides and plastics. Because of the possibility of a mass toxic exposure, public health officials began a detailed investigation. The end result of the investigation itself would prove a great surprise.

It was eventually discovered that the urine of a number of children without symptoms tested positive for n-butylbenzine sulfonamide—and the chemical itself was eventually traced to the inside surface of the plastic containers used to collect the urine samples. Urine samples collected in glass containers showed no trace of the chemical.

Finally, it appeared that there was one single factor linked to the student's having become ill, which was that they had observed another child developing symptoms first. Despite that fact, many East Templeton residents continue to believe that the children suffered from toxic exposure.

The East Templeton case was eventually reported in a medical journal, and the facts we have just reviewed are exactly as published. There have also been numerous reports of medical mass hysteria in the workplace. This time, let's construct a composite story demonstrating what most of these events have in common.

A few employees in an office or factory smell a nasty odor. A rumor starts that some toxic fumes have been accidentally released. Meanwhile, one or two workers faint or complain of severe headache and nausea. Soon, other workers are all complaining of headaches and nausea, and some are fainting. The day could end with thirty or forty workers in the local emergency room all suffering from the same symptoms. Later, after a full investigation occurs, the source of the odor is located and it turns out to be something offensive but totally harmless. (Hahn states that one well-documented case of mass hysteria ended up involving more than nine hundred people.)

When the investigation is concluded, it often turns out the first few workers to be afflicted suffer from existing health difficulties probably responsible for the symptoms, which have little if anything to do with the "fumes." The other workers, observing their coworkers becoming ill while also smelling the fumes, participate in a "negative expectation chain reaction." Naturally, the more people developing symptoms, the more powerful the suggestion that something is terribly wrong, making it even more likely that still more workers will succumb.

We've now seen enough to be convinced that the nocebo effect is almost certainly real. Now let's discuss how best to classify it.

The Nocebo Effect: Has It Earned a Name of Its Own?

If our meaning model is correct, then whenever a patient is treated the way Patty was treated by Dr. Graubert, we'd expect a positive placebo response would likely occur. When a patient sees a physician or nurse and feels less listened to, without a good explanation, uncared for, and less in control, then we'd predict that a nocebo effect is possible. This means that in our complex and too often impersonal health care system, nocebo effects must be rather common.

Do we actually need "nocebo" as a stand-alone phenomenon? Answering this will depend on future research which may reveal the bodily mechanisms that produce it. We've already seen that Dr. Hahn attributes the nocebo effect, at the level of the mind, to the same mechanism to which many attribute the placebo response: the person's expectations. In the next chapter, we'll review the various chemical pathways by which the placebo response might operate. If future research shows that the chemical pathways that account for nocebo effects are completely different from those that produce positive placebo responses, then we'll be fully justified in keeping two different terms for the two different reactions.

My own guess is that we will find mostly the same pathways involved because, as we will see, each of the pathways is capable of producing either a lot, or too little, of the healing products it is responsible for. I'd be willing to bet that in Patty's case, the same chemical pathway, the stress pathway, was involved in her reaction to each phone call: increasing after talking to Sheila Garrison, and then decreasing after talking with Dr. Graubert. If that is true, then I advocate keeping a single term, the placebo response. As we have defined placebo response, it is what happens when a change occurs in the body as a result of altered symbolic significance. The definition is open to this change being either for the better or for the worse.

In the chapters that follow, we'll have limited need to use the concept of nocebo. This is especially true because our later focus will be on what you yourself can do to promote your own healing, so of course we will be much more interested in positive than in negative changes. The nocebo effect is still very important, however, because it adds to the scientific evidence that expectancy can produce bodily changes.

NINE

From Meaning to Bodily Change: The Biochemical Pathways

"Nobody has yet devised an experiment to show the effect on rats of living my life."

—Ashleigh Brilliant

We've now seen that the placebo response can be produced by what we expect and by our past experiences with healing. We've also observed that these expectations and recollections affect our minds by the meaning that we attach to the experience of being ill. The stories we tell ourselves and each other about illness are our main method of attaching meaning to these situations. We now have to complete the scientific picture of the placebo response by following the mind-body sequence of events to its conclusion.

You've already been introduced to the concept of pathways of the body, a term scientists often use to describe a series of causes and effects. We'll be concentrating here on those pathways which begin with a change in the meaning of the illness experience, and end with a change in how we feel or how our body functions. The biochemical substances produced as a result of activating these pathways are the scientific correlate of what we have been calling, in general terms, the body's "inner pharmacy."

Science has yet to discover a single pathway that accounts for the placebo response. What we know about the uncertainties and variations in the response makes the most sense if we imagine that sometimes the placebo response works by one pathway, and sometimes by another. Our inner pharmacies, it would seem, have quite an array of different biochemical substances on their shelves. In this chapter, I will concentrate on three known mind-body healing pathways and point out the unique features of each one. These features are exactly what will lead us to a scientific accounting of how the placebo response could ignite our inner pharmacies.

Let's begin our discussion of the placebo response pathways by thinking about modern ideas of brain anatomy and brain chemistry, starting with a comparison of classical reductionism and the new neuroscience.

Meaning and Brain Chemistry

Reductionism assumes that we cannot really comprehend anything which happens to an object unless it can be understood in terms of the measurable behavior of the smaller pieces that comprise it—ideally, molecules and atoms. Although reductionistic thinking has long been popular in many branches of science and medicine, psychiatry has recently become one of its most fertile fields. Under the banner of "biological psychiatry," many practitioners have dismissed all concern with meaning and consciousness, focusing instead on chemicals in the brain.

Biological psychiatry does indeed seem a concept whose time has come: For many years, psychoanalytic psychiatrists—who tried "talk therapy" on people with such severe mental diseases as schizophrenia, depression, and manic-depressive disorder—achieved only limited success. Beginning in the 1950s, new drugs were introduced to treat these disorders and the difference between their effectiveness against these disorders and the old "talk" approach was quite striking. The molecular cure certainly appeared to be much more powerful and satisfying than the talk cure. So psychiatrists could perhaps be forgiven if they concluded, "Forget what the patient is thinking, and what this experience means to him; just find out which molecules are malfunctioning in which brain location, and find a way to fix them."

Because of the popularity of biological psychiatry and the fact that some of its recent success stories (for instance, Prozac for depression) have been widely touted in the popular media, it is especially important to point out that the best thinking in modern neuroscience is going in quite a different direction. Moreover, we should be aware that some critics of biological psychiatric treatment argue that when you carefully assess the evidence, many modern psychiatric medicines are really not proven to be any better than placebos. This brand of modern neuroscience is just as interested in brain scans, precise anatomic location of brain processes, and molecular reactions as reductionism—but, at the same time, doesn't dismiss meaning or consciousness.

To the reductionist, the placebo response always has been and always will be a mystery. Milk sugar (lactose), taken in the form of a pill, so far as we know has no measurable biochemical effect on the brain, or on the rest of the body for that matter. So why should it relieve pain? By contrast, to the best modern version of neuroscience, it would be quite surprising if the placebo response did *not* occur. After all, if the patient attributes some meaning to taking the placebo pill, then the following sequence is set in motion:

1. If the patient thinks differently, then the chemistry of the brain must undergo a change, because consciousness and brain chemistry are correlated.
2. If brain chemistry undergoes a change, then certain other biochemical pathways which link the brain to the rest of the body could undergo changes as well.
3. If those brain-body pathways undergo changes, then the tissues of the body which are influenced by those pathways could also be changed.
4. If the bodily tissues are changed by those biochemical influences, then healing might occur.

Now, the question remains: Can we identify any of those biochemical pathways?

As I mentioned earlier, three pathways seem to suggest promise. I say "suggest" because there is still scant proof that the pathways are altered when patients take placebos or when the placebo response is triggered in some other fashion. Regrettably, most of the researchers whose work I've been reporting do not measure these biochemical pathways. Consequently, we have virtually no data directly linking any understanding of meaning and symbolic significance with biochemistry. Dr. David McClelland's Mother Teresa experiment was an interesting exception. Instead, we have general evidence that three biochemical pathways are easily influenced by other mental and conscious processes. This makes them good places to look when we finally do the experiments necessary to link meaning with biochemistry.

The Endorphin Pathways

Compare a list of drugs commonly used by physicians in 1800 with a list of drugs used today. There will be only a handful that appear on both lists—and one of them is the opium family of narcotic painkillers. Despite decades of scientific research, medicine has discovered no drug that works better for severe pain than morphine and other close cousins or derivatives of opium.

Recently, scientists have begun to understand better how such drugs as opium derivatives influence the body's cells. The outer surface or envelope of the cell, the cell membrane, is a very complex chemical structure that contains special areas called receptors. The shape of the molecules that make up the receptor area match the patterns of other molecules which might turn up in the cell's environment. Sometimes it's convenient to think of receptors as a sort of "parking place" for molecules on the cell's surface, but each receptor allows only a particular molecular "car," not just any "car," to park there.

When a molecule floats by the right receptor, they link together much like two adjacent pieces of a jigsaw puzzle, assuring that only a particular molecule will be able to bind to any particular receptor site on the cell membrane. Also, only certain sorts of cells will have receptors for certain molecules. This explains why a chemical—a drug or a hormone or other chemical messenger from the body itself—might have a major effect on certain cells, but no effect at all on other kinds.

The binding of the outside molecule to the receptor then causes the cell's internal chemical factory to begin making new substances, which in turn alter the cell's function. This means the outside molecule has the power to change how the cell behaves without actually going inside it. Usually, after an appropriate period of time, the cell receptor lets go of the outside molecule and allows it to float away again. This disengagement turns off the inner chemical factory, causing the cell to return to the way it was before.

The receptor sites on the membranes of different cells allow the body to regulate how all of its tissues and organs function. The body has a wide array of traveling messenger molecules which can turn on or turn off the processes inside various cells, and the receptor-molecule fit assures that the message will be received only by the correct cell. We now understand that many drugs given by physicians are effective because they can bind to cell membrane receptors. Often this happens when the molecule of the drug happens to be shaped very much like the portion of the body's naturally occurring molecule-messenger for that cell, so that it fits the jigsaw puzzle pattern well enough to bind to the cell membrane. As we'll see, this turns out to be the case with drugs like morphine.

Scientists first discovered that human brain cells have receptors which seem especially designed to react to molecules of morphine and other opium-like compounds. These receptor sites helped explain why this class of drugs works so well to control pain. A little more searching revealed the reason these receptors exist in the body: The body makes its own messenger molecules which, in their chemical structure, happen to look a lot like morphine, and bind to the same cell receptors. These "inside (the body) morphine" substances were named *endorphins.*

Later studies showed that endorphins in brain tissue were related to relief of pain. Extra endorphins could even cause euphoria, a high similar to taking addictive drugs. Some have proposed that runners and weight lifters experience an endorphin high, which could explain why running or working out becomes akin to an addiction. Scientists were able to identify specific portions of the brain where endorphins are manufactured, the periaqueductal gray matter and rostroventral medulla regions being especially important. Electrical stimulation of the periaqueductal gray matter of a rat made the cells there secrete more endorphin. Researchers could then do a major operation on the rat's belly, with the rat completely awake yet showing no sign of pain. There was one practical problem with studying endorphins in humans, a concept medical scientists call the blood-brain barrier. Most of our bodies' organs are in fairly easy communication with the bloodstream. For example, we can tell that a patient has had a heart attack by putting a needle in the vein of the arm, taking a sample of circulating blood, and running tests on it. When heart muscle is damaged, certain chemicals are released that go directly into the bloodstream, float through the entire circulation, and can easily be measured in any blood sample.

The brain is in a more protected state, probably for sound safety reasons, so it's much harder for molecules inside it to pass into the body's blood supply, and even more difficult for chemicals circulating in the blood to enter and affect brain tissue. Because endorphins work mostly inside the brain tissue, it's also difficult to measure endorphin levels in blood samples to get reliable estimates of how much endorphin is being released. When experimenting on rats, you can find out about endorphin levels by taking a sample of tissue from the rat's brain. For obvious reasons, this is usually not possible in experiments on humans. Subsequently, many studies of endorphins had to rely upon very indirect measurements.

This is what happened in the first study that set out to link the placebo response to endorphins. Drs. Jon Levine, Newton Gordon, and Howard Fields of the University of California, San Francisco, took advantage of a fact previously shown in other research. A drug called naloxone is a morphine antagonist, blocking or stopping its effects. Since it is sufficiently similar to the morphine jigsaw puzzle piece, naloxone can bind very solidly to the morphine cell receptor; yet it is sufficiently dissimilar from morphine not to cause the cell to behave differently in its internal chemical function. The naloxone molecule does not make the cell do whatever it needs to do to relieve the pain sensation; but by taking up the morphine parking place, the naloxone prevents the morphine from doing its work. This is of great benefit when a patient is in danger of dying from an overdose of morphine. A shot of naloxone will reverse the symptoms of overdose within minutes.

Since endorphins are so closely allied to morphine in their chemical structure, we might expect that naloxone would do to endorphins exactly what it does to morphine. And so it seemed, at least at the time that Dr. Levine and his colleagues did their study some twenty years ago. Naloxone had previously been shown in a number of experiments to be a potent blocker of the effects of endorphins, so Levine's team decided to run a test of their own.

The scientists gathered together a group of patients suffering from wisdom tooth extraction and gave them placebo injections. Some of the subjects received a shot of naloxone; some did not. Levine and his colleagues noted that a number of them, as expected, reported a reduction in pain after the placebo injection; but those subjects who got the naloxone injection reported that their pain returned much more quickly. From that data, it seemed that whatever good the placebo did was undone by the naloxone. Drs. Levine, Gordon, and Fields reported that, with this circumstantial evidence, they had shown that the placebo pain relief must have been caused by the release of endorphins in the brain.

There was great excitement at Levine's report, though only some of it was warranted. The findings provided the first linkage between the use of a placebo and a biochemical pathway inside the body that could, at least in theory, explain how the placebo achieved its effects. But there was an overreading of the importance of Levine's findings. Many reports stated, "We finally understand how placebos work."

We have seen that placebos do a lot more than relieve pain. They can lower blood pressure in hypertension, lower blood sugar in diabetes, and perhaps even on occasion cause shrinkage in malignant tumors, to cite only a few examples. Since there is no reason today to believe that endorphins are involved in all of those processes, linking endorphins to placebos in pain relief is hardly an explanation of *all* placebo responses.

There is another limitation to the research, which was not appreciated by many medical commentators. Knowing that endorphins are involved in placebo pain relief does not explain why some patients given placebos seem to release endorphins and others do not. In order to understand this difference, we need to grasp the meaning that each individual attaches to the experience of having the pain and taking the placebo. If we could measure each person's resulting endorphin levels, and tie those data together with data about the meaning each person attaches to the experience, then we would indeed have a very solid explanation of how placebos work, at least in pain relief. As long as we look only at endorphins and not at meaning or symbolic significance, we have only half the story—an interesting and challenging half, perhaps, but still only half.

Later research both by Levine's team and by others showed that the situation was even more complicated. First, additional studies were unable to show a completely consistent pattern of pain increase or decrease when placebos were followed by naloxone. Second, additional research suggested that naloxone itself was a more complicated substance than was originally thought, seeming to have the actual power to make the pain worse without affecting the action of endorphins. This observation cast doubt on the assumption that we could know how the endorphins were working by watching the response to naloxone.

The most significant suppositions came from new discoveries about different endorphin pathways or systems. Scientists now believe that there are at least five different types of endorphins and three different endorphin receptors. Some of the endorphin receptors appear to be clustered in the brain. Their existence explains how pain is relieved when one takes medicines which are absorbed into it. Other receptors appear to be clustered in parts of the spinal cord, and their discovery shows how spinal and epidural anesthesia may work.

At any rate, we can appreciate that the endorphin system is itself

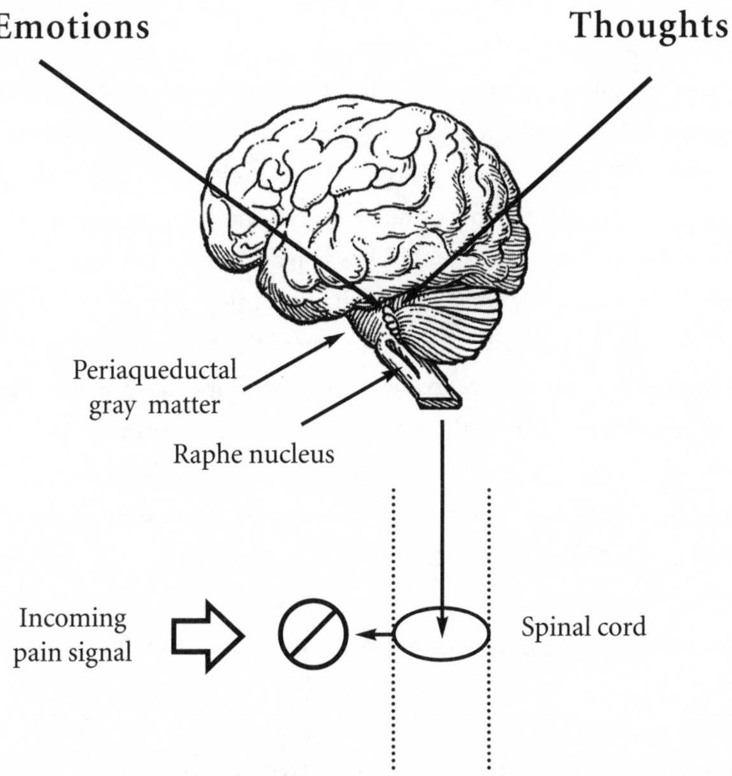

Brain cells that secrete endorphins include those in the periaqueductal gray matter and those in the rostroventral medulla, near the raphe nucleus. The periaqueductal gray matter is located in a portion of the brain that is richly supplied with connections from other brain centers responsible for emotions and thought. Some nerve cells form a direct bridge between the periaqueductal gray matter and the raphe nucleus. Cells beginning at the raphe nucleus, in turn, run down the spinal cord and connect to a portion of the cord that is also capable of secreting endorphins. As a result of turning on these nerve pathways, by the secretion of endorphins, incoming pain signals approaching the spinal cord (which normally transmits pain messages from the rest of the body up to the brain) are diminished or blocked.

extremely complicated. Simply to say that placebos work to relieve pain by turning on the endorphin pathway is quite inadequate as a scientific explanation. We may eventually learn that some placebo responses involve certain endorphin molecules which attach to certain receptor sites, while different placebo responses involve different endorphin molecules which do their work at different sites.

You will recall from chapter 6 the two-armed experimental design developed by Dr. Nicholas Voudouris and then later used by Guy Montgomery and Dr. Irving Kirsch. Montgomery and Kirsch reasoned that everything we know about endorphins suggests that they are a general and not a local phenomenon. That is, if the way placebos work is by triggering the release of endorphins, this ought to have as much impact on the right arm as upon the left arm, or any other part of the body. They concluded that in their experiment, placebos reduced pain, but could not have done so by release of endorphins. Whatever happened in their subjects was quite localized to the region where the placebo cream was applied.

Here is another possibility: While some of the body's endorphin receptors are clustered in the brain, others are clustered in the spinal cord. If we expect pain relief on the left arm but not on the right, perhaps the left side of the spinal cord is stimulated to secrete endorphins while the right side isn't. This reinforces the point that the endorphin system is what scientists call a descending neural pathway. That is, the endophin system starts in the brain but travels downward through the spinal cord and eventually through the peripheral nerves to affect one specific spot on the surface of the body. Animal experiments show that if you cut some of those nerve pathways in the spinal cord, the brain endorphins may fail to relieve pain. Some endorphin pain relief may be in the brain and affect the whole body at once, while other effects of the endorphin pathways may be very localized.

Probably the best answer today to the placebo-endorphin question is that we have a strong suspicion that at least some placebo pain relief, and perhaps the effects placebos have on anxiety and shortness of breath, occur because placebos stimulate the release of endorphins. But exactly which endorphin pathway is involved, and at what sites within the brain or the nervous system, remains a mystery.

One recent study represents perhaps the best evidence supporting an endorphin mechanism, and showing the complexity of the placebo response. Drs. Martina Amanzio and Fabrizio Benedetti of Torino, Italy, performed an extremely complicated experiment in the psychology laboratory on placebo pain relief. Using expectancy and conditioning, they found that both produced some placebo response and that combined, they produced an even more substantial response.

Drs. Amanzio and Benedetti did find that if the placebo response was produced by expectancy only, it was completely eliminated by giving naloxone. When they gave naloxone all by itself, it did not change the pain level in their subjects. If the response was produced solely by conditioning, response to naloxone depended upon which drug was used as the unconditioned stimulus. If they conditioned the subjects using morphine, then giving the naloxone eliminated the placebo response. If they used ketorolac (Toradol), a pain-killing drug completely unrelated to the morphine and opium family, naloxone had no effect on the conditioning-induced placebo response.

They concluded that when placebo pain relief is induced by expectancy, it is probably a result of activation of an endorphin pathway. When the placebo response is produced by conditioning, the precise pathway depends upon the specific chemical substance used for the conditioning.

Let's consider a second system with an enormous effect on how we feel, both physically and emotionally: the stress pathway.

The Stress/Relaxation Response

The stress pathway is the oldest example in twentieth century medical science of linking biochemistry with the mind, yet there are few, if any, studies which tie it directly to the placebo response. No survey of the potential biochemical pathways that connect changes in meaning with changes in the body's health can omit mention of the stress pathway, because:

- The biochemical stress pathway has proven itself, over many decades, to be exquisitely sensitive to changes in the state of the mind; and

- The biochemical stress pathway has also revealed itself to be implicated in a number of disease processes, including:

- Hypertension
- Hardening of the arteries
- Heart attacks
- Osteoporosis
- Memory loss
- Accelerated aging
- Stomach ulcers
- Fibromyalgia (a chronic pain condition)
- Chronic fatigue syndrome
- Eczema
- Vulnerability to infections

Therefore, if in the future we ever see an Institute of the Placebo Response established to conduct thorough, integrated research into all aspects of the phenomenon, then the studies would necessarily include investigation of the stress pathway as a very likely "suspect" for playing a major role in the inner pharmacy.

Obviously, the stress pathway is turned on or off by the level of stress the individual experiences. We should agree on a basic definition of stress, because today we commonly regard it quite differently from the view proposed by the pioneer biologists who studied the stress pathway. Stress to us encompasses such disparate events as how the boss treats us at work and arguing with teenage children over who gets the car. But these examples are not bodily reactions; they're signals from the environment which could produce a stress reaction in our bodies. Biologists would want to be precise and term these outside signals and events *stressors*. They would then reserve the term "stress" to describe the changes produced in our bodies when we are exposed to stressors.

Let's take a detailed look at the stress pathway.

- Such brain areas as the amygdala and the hippocampus are very sensitive to emotional changes. They are also connected with the thinking centers of the brain in the cortex, so that how we think

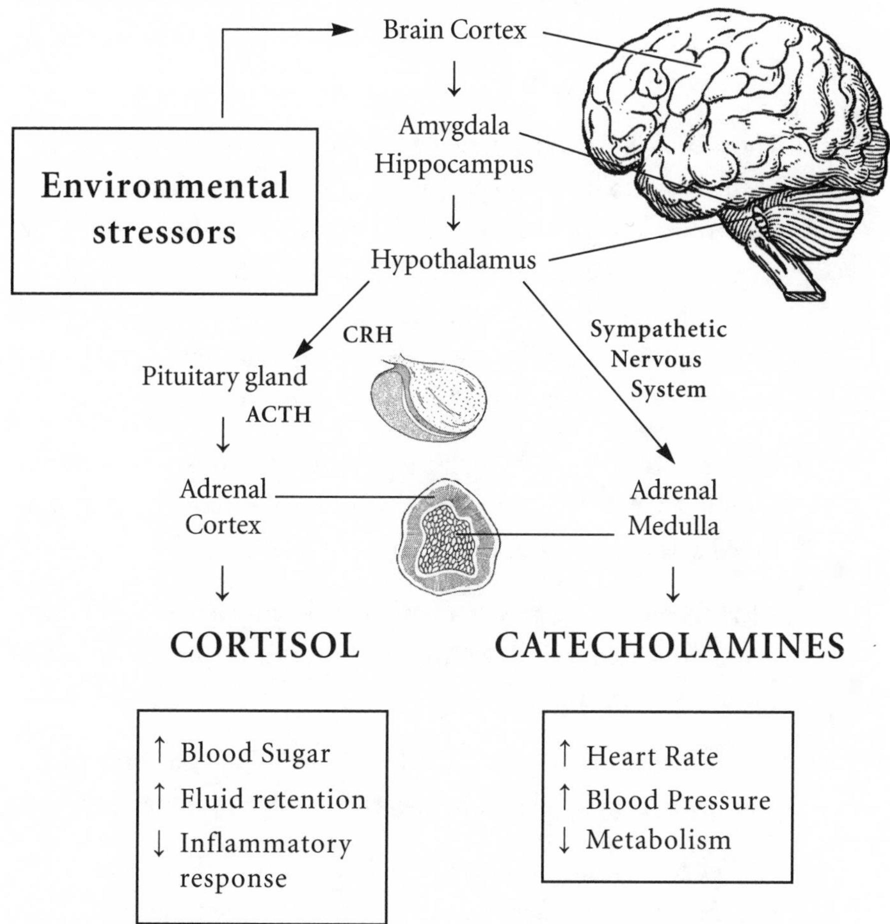

Stress/Relaxation Pathway

When the brain cortex perceives environmental stressors, it sends nerve impulses to the hypothalamus, passing on the way the amygdala and hippocampus, portions of the brain involved in emotional states. From the hypothalamus, two pathways emerge. In one, corticotropin-releasing hormone (CRH) is secreted, which causes the pituitary gland to make more adrenocorticotropic hormone (ACTH). ACTH in turn acts on the outer portion of the adrenal gland, the adrenal cortex, to manufacture more of the hormone cortisol. The other pathway from the hypothalamus sends nerve impulses via the sympathetic nervous system to the inner portion of the adrenal gland, the adrenal medulla, where the manufacture of catecholamines occurs. A *stress response* is the result when there is an increase in cortisol and catecholamines; when these substances are decreased, a *relaxation resonse* occurs instead.

about events—including the meaning that we attach to events, or the stories we tell about events—will influence the reaction of these emotional centers.

- Those brain areas are intimately connected with an area at the base of the brain called the hypothalamus. The hypothalamus is a very important crossroads because it lies outside the blood-brain barrier we spoke of earlier. This means that other chemicals circulating in the bloodstream, including ones entering from the environment, can influence it. So the hypothalamus is extremely sensitive both to our mental states and to outside factors.
- The hypothalamus, when it's stimulated by stressors, performs several different tasks. One of them is to make more of a hormone called corticotropin-releasing hormone (CRH).
- CRH then takes a very short trip to the front part of the pituitary gland, which dangles down from the base of the brain just below the hypothalamus.
- When turned on by CRH, the front part of the pituitary makes another hormone called adrenocorticotropic hormone or ACTH.
- ACTH has to take a longer trip, because it goes by way of the bloodstream from the pituitary gland to the adrenal glands, which sit on top of the kidneys.
- The outer portion of the adrenal gland (called the adrenal cortex), when stimulated by ACTH, manufactures the steroid hormone called cortisol.
- Cortisol is one of the body's master hormones because it has several important effects on a wide variety of cells. For example, it raises blood sugar levels; it causes the body to retain salt and fluids; and it reduces the body's inflammatory and immune responses.

Sometimes body pathways have branches, and the stress pathway has an important one.

- As the hypothalamus makes more CRH when it senses stress, it also stimulates heightened electrical signals in the nerve pathways called the sympathetic nervous system. This system is part of the autonomic nerve system of the body, as it deals with things like heartbeat and breathing that go on automatically without our ever being aware of them. In this way, a change in the meaning of an event, which could be consciously perceived in the higher parts of the brain, turns into unconscious events in the body.

- The nerve pathways of the sympathetic nervous system end up in a different portion of the adrenal gland, the inner portion or adrenal medulla. There they cause the gland to make more of a class of substances called catecholamines, the best known of which is epinephrine, or adrenaline.

- Catecholamines act vigorously on the heart and blood vessels, causing increased heart rate and blood pressure, more rapid breathing, and a faster metabolic rate throughout the body.

- The sympathetic nervous system also influences our muscular network, generally increasing muscle tension and rigidity. In the short term, this can prepare us for the fight or flight response; if kept up over the long haul, it can greatly worsen musculoskeletal pain problems like low back pain and tension headache.

Many decades ago, the stress pathway was shown to produce the fight or flight response both in animals and humans: A high epinephrine level causes the heart to beat faster, blood pressure to go up, faster breathing, and sweating; and a high cortisol level makes more sugar available to the blood for bolstered energy. Essentially, the stress response does what is necessary to prepare the animal or the person either to fight or to run if threatened by danger. The opposite reaction, which Dr. Herbert Benson calls the "relaxation response," occurs when the level of epinephrine and other catecholamines drops below normal.

We know that the symptoms associated with anxiety or panic attacks are precisely those which are linked to a high catecholamine level. We also know that some people who seem to be chronically anxious tend to have high catecholamine levels most of the time. Their bodies secrete an amount of catecholamines which in a less tense person would be associated with a high state of arousal—only for these anxious people, the body seems to think that this is its normal state and should be maintained all day, every day. And we know further that people who have these chronically high catecholamine levels are more prone to certain diseases, especially heart disease, high blood pressure, and ulcer disease.

Dr. Benson, in his book *The Relaxation Response,* has also shown that these diseases can be prevented with a variety of simple exercises which can dramatically lower catecholamine levels in anxious and normal people. He has shown how a number of common practices in many cultures, many religious rituals, for example, are actually forms of these relaxation exercises, demonstrating how human culture has evolved over millennia to save us from the dangers of too much stress.

Dr. Dean Ornish has also shown us how to prevent further heart attacks in people with serious coronary artery disease—and even how to open up their blocked coronary arteries—without the use of drugs. The Ornish program contains a number of elements, among them a very low-fat diet and moderate exercise, that work principally on the fats in our bloodstream. But it also includes such elements as the same moderate exercise, yoga and meditation, and social support that probably act on the stress pathway, even though the bloodstream fat level and the catecholamine level are somewhat linked. His program overall is fat-lowering and stress-lowering.

When Dr. Ornish started his work, he thought that bringing together groups of heart-disease sufferers was incidental to the rest of the program: It was simply more efficient to explain the diet and to teach yoga techniques to a roomful of people instead of individually. He later came to believe that the group activities themselves were an extremely important part of the success of the program.

We've already discussed the importance of social support in triggering the inner pharmacy. Dr. Ornish and other scientists and physicians bear out this concept by showing the very dramatic effect of social support and social isolation on risk of heart disease, with socially isolated people having a two to four times higher risk of dying of heart disease than people with good social support.

To summarize this area of research, do we have any clues how to look for the mysterious links between the stress pathway and the placebo response?

First, the social isolation example might lead us to think that the care and concern element of the meaning model might be especially closely linked with this biochemical pathway. If we recall the example of the doulas in labor, and the case of Dr. Shaw and her Indian friend, we can imagine how the stress levels of the women might have increased as a result of being alone, and how having a calm, and calming, companion could dramatically reduce the stress level. Research has demonstrated that high catecholamine levels in labor can slow down its course and decrease the amount of blood going to the baby, thus producing a higher likelihood of medical complications.

Second, when we are looking at the placebo response in diseases which are known to be linked to the stress pathway, we might especially want to measure cortisol and catecholamine levels to see if reducing them is inherent in placebo response.

Since so many different diseases have all been shown to be related to the stress pathway, proven linkage between this pathway and the placebo response could help to explain why the placebo response has been shown to affect such a wide variety of conditions.

Third, we could investigate further the link between the meaning the person assigns to the illness or symptom, the level of cortisol or catecholamines released, and the resultant bodily changes. We know that the stress response is exquisitely sensitive to meaning. In the case of Patty and her "medical hexing," we can imagine that she underwent a radically heightened stress response when the nurse told her that her bleeding might be cancer, and she experienced a significant relaxation response when she spoke with her reassuring internist.

Similarly, if we interpret a symptom as a sign of impeding danger or doom, we will have one level of stress response. If we attach a new meaning to the same symptom, so that we see it merely as a nuisance, we will have a totally different level of stress response. In the end, this could help to solve the puzzle of why many symptoms respond well to placebos and the reassurance provided by the encounter with the physician or other healer.

A number of older studies have suggested that the best placebo responders are people with a moderate level of anxiety when they first see the physician. Those with very high anxiety, or with no anxiety, do not respond as well. This is what we should expect if we imagine that one aspect of the placebo response in the body is the lowering of cortisol and catecholamine levels. If they were very low to start with, we would not be able to detect a placebo response. If levels were extremely high, the amount of lowering produced by the placebo response might not be sufficient to reduce other symptoms.

Psychoneuroimmune Pathways

This area of research is relatively new and has caused great excitement among those interested in mind-body medicine. My impression of its current state is that it has proven, beyond reasonable doubt, that mental and emotional changes can alter the immune system. What has not yet been proven is that these changes are truly important, or can be harnessed, in the causation or prevention of disease. It may well be so; but the research so far has been preliminary, not conclusive.

The name psychoneuroimmunology first appeared as a title of a book in 1981, and was developed by Robert Ader, whose work on conditioning we reviewed in chapter 6. The term signaled a better understanding of the relationship between the immune system and other bodily functions. Until then, the immune system had been seen by scientists as independent of most of the rest of the body, existing for one purpose only: to recognize, and then to attack, foreign substances which might enter the body and cause disease.

The old theory says that when the immune system works correctly, it is activated by the appearance of some foreign particle like a virus. If it works incorrectly—attacking healthy tissues of the body itself, in such autoimmune diseases as rheumatoid arthritis—then perhaps it is triggered at first by an overreaction to a virus or other foreign invasion; or perhaps the attack on the bodily tissues is purely random and uncontrollable. One thing seems clear: The regulatory systems that operate on other parts of the body, especially the conscious mind, are powerless over the immune system.

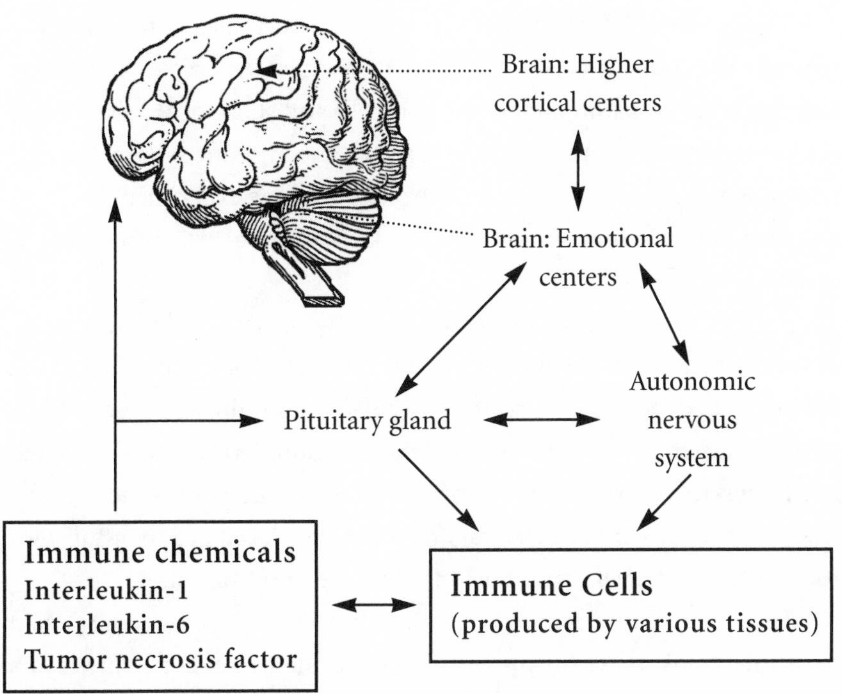

Psychoneuroimmune Pathways

Schematic diagram of communication linkages between the immune system and other body systems. The immune cells act as a sensory organ, sending messages about the state of the body and the environment back to the brain. The brain, in turn, acting in part through the other pathways described in this chapter, influences the manufacture and function of immune cells (adapted from Figure 1.2 in Alan Watkins, "Mind-Body Pathways," in *Mind-Body Medicine: A Clinician's Guide to Psychoneuroimmunology,* edited by Alan Watkins (New York: Churchill Livingston, 1997).

What psychoneuroimmunology has taught us is that the grand independence of the immune system is a myth. As it turns out, various tissues in which immune cells and substances are manufactured are richly supplied with nerve endings. Immune cells are studded with receptor sites for molecules that are released as a result of nervous system changes. Some of these neuropeptide molecules, which have special receptor sites, or parking places, on the surfaces of the immune cells, are known to be precisely those neuropeptides whose levels rise and fall with changes in emotional state.

The exchange of information between the nervous and immune systems works in both directions. Not only do changes in nervous stimulation alter the types and amounts of immune cells and substances produced by the body, but when something else turns on the immune system, the nervous system responds with changes of its own. One experiment showing this may illustrate how some of the work in psychoneuroimmunology is carried out.

A virus called "Newcastle virus" typically causes no obvious disease in rats. In fact, the animals infected with the virus continue as if nothing has happened. Some investigators decided to administer doses of the virus to rats and then, a few hours later, measure levels of stress-related hormones in several portions of the animals' nervous systems. The response proved similar to the rats' having been placed in a stressful environment, receiving electric shocks to their feet, for example.

The investigators pointed out that even if the Newcastle virus had been infectious, these hormone changes seemed to occur many hours before actual symptoms of disease could have developed. Their explanation was that the initial ignition of the immune system in response to the virus invasion—which, they suspected, was the release of an immune chemical called interleukin-1—sent a message to the animal's nervous system that something potentially stressful was happening. The rest of the animal's systems rose to a heightened level of alertness. The hypothalamus seems to be especially sensitive to incoming signals from the immune system.

Some scientists have suggested that the body might have an ideal level of stress response for keeping the immune system at its optimal state. If the hypothalamus and the pituitary gland produce too little of some of their products, perhaps the body is more prone to autoimmune diseases. On the other hand, if these products are constantly at too high a level, the individual may be more prone to addictions, panic disorders, and chronic conditions like cancer. Some investigators add further that exactly where the "set point" is for the ideal level of hypothalamic-pituitary function for each individual might be genetically determined. This could explain why emotional states, lifestyle, and inherited tendencies all seem to influence who is at risk for certain diseases.

Psychoneuroimmunology also seems to explain why people who have undergone stressful life changes, like the death of a loved one, severe depression, or divorce, seem to be more prone to disease. It also turns out to be a point of intersection among all three of the possible placebo pathways we have looked at in this chapter. That is, endorphin release and cortisol and catecholamine levels are also part of the body's natural reaction to stressful changes, and these substances are part of the psychoneuroimmune feedback system and can alter immune function which, in turn, can be further altered themselves by immune system changes. Perhaps, we have a solid theory for solving an aspect of the mystery: The three pathways we have listed are really one grand, interconnected pathway.

Now, having discovered some tantalizing clues, we need to throw a little cold water on the proceedings. For all its advances, psychoneuroimmunology has not yet produced many of the remarkable gains it first promised. As I said at the beginning of this section, it has proven to be relatively easy to measure differences in immune function that correlate with various alterations in the nervous system or the person's emotional state or behavior. But linking those immune system changes with the actual cause or cure of human diseases has been much harder.

Even when you have designed a treatment approach that actually helps sick people, it may be very hard to prove that it works by psychoneuroimmunological pathways. One example will illustrate some of this complexity. Dr. Fawzy Fawzy and his colleagues at UCLA were able to design one of the most helpful psychological tools to assist patients who had recently undergone surgery for malignant melanoma. They found that their six-week program of counseling and support groups helped the patients cope better with the aftermath of surgery and cancer treatment. Not only that, but the patients who attended the support group survived longer, on average, than a control group who did not. One would think their support-group attendees would be an ideal experimental group to demonstrate how altered immune function might link the psychological support with the enhanced survival.

Dr. Fawzy and colleagues did indeed find something very impressive when they looked at the immune functions of his subjects at the end of the six-week program, and then again six months later. They discovered some fairly isolated immune changes at six weeks, but much more impressive immune changes at six months. Included in the six-month changes was an increase in the number of natural killer cells, a type of immune cell thought to be especially important in warding off cancer spread. Thus, they concluded that the impact of the six-week program was indeed long-term.

The problem, however, was that no direct link could be shown between any of these immune changes and important measures of cancer progression. For example, those subjects who had more of the natural killer cells at six months showed fewer cancer recurrences; but surprisingly, this was not linked statistically to longer survival. So Dr. Fawzy was very careful to explain that he had designed a helpful form of support group, which produced long-lasting changes, but that he had been unable directly to link those psychological support changes to specific disease outcomes by means of the immune system.

And so another aspect of our mystery remains unsolved, at least so far. Perhaps, a future experiment will provide evidence of the linkages that Fawzy's group was unable to prove.

For our purposes in this chapter, we need not worry too much about what has or has not been proven in this field. All we are doing, after all, is listing potential linkages that might explain placebo responses. The fact that the immune system undergoes changes attributable to what we think and feel about what is going on around us, gives us a potential clue as to one means by which a placebo response might work. At the very least, instead of thinking the immune system is separate from the effects of the mind, we need to remember that it seems designed specifically to influence and to be influenced by both the mind and the nervous system.

Future Research: The Promise of Imaging

The best modern neuroscience has shown us two very important things. First, when our minds change in some way, the chemistry in our brains changes correspondingly. We should expect that changes in brain chemistry could ultimately lead to changes in the function of other processes elsewhere in the body. Second, as we've discussed, our sense organs are constantly being barraged by signals from the environment: changing sights, sounds, and smells.

A healthy life requires a number of built-in filters which enable the person to ignore the great majority of signals, which are simply noise, and to pay attention to the relatively few that really matter. The human brain is especially constructed to focus on *meanings and relationships* in sorting out which signals to attend to. When we construct meanings to explain things that happen to us, and when we are involved in such important, ongoing human relationships as our relationships with physicians and other healers, then those signals are given priority status when they are picked up by the body's sense organs. The human body seems to be hardwired to take meaningful signals from the environment and translate these into changes in bodily processes which can lead to healing.

Though research into the placebo response ought to continue in many areas using many different methods, perhaps the next major advances will come from the application of brain imaging. Positron emission tomography (PET) scanners and special variations of magnetic resonance imaging (MRI) scans are allowing medical scientists to "see" inside the human brain.

This technology allows scientists to see which centers of a person's brain, at any given moment, are chemically most active. This suggests which brain cells are busy firing off electrical signals. Because the person remains awake before, during, and after the scanning process, it's easy to get the person to describe what thoughts or impressions are going on at the same time. In this way, brain anatomy and brain chemistry can be correlated with thoughts and emotions, as well as with whatever signals were sent to the person as the scan was taken.

Consider some further uses for these scans. When we discussed expectancy theory, we noted that some psychologists see two sets of brain circuits involved: bottom-up circuits bringing information in from the environment ("The nurse just gave me a shot"), and top-down circuits holding stored information from past experiences ("When I get a shot, I usually feel better afterward"). If scans could be done immediately after patients take a medication, or otherwise receive a healing signal from the environment, we might not have to speculate on the nature and location of these circuits; we might be able to see precisely which brain circuits are being activated. And if, out of ten subjects, five experienced a placebo response and five did not, we might see whether the scans of the responders differed in any reproducible way from the scans of the nonresponders.

These scans would provide valuable clues of an additional sort. Scientists know that cells in different parts of the brain tend to secrete different chemicals. Noting that a certain brain location has lit up on the scan might be a tip-off that the neuropeptide or other chemical made there is now being secreted. This might provide clues as to which chemical pathways are then responsible for whatever placebo response may later occur. For example, we noted that the periaqueductal gray area is one of the regions especially involved in endorphin secretion. If a scan showed particularly high chemical activity in the periaqueductal gray region, this could be helpful circumstantial evidence that whatever bodily changes occurred later on might be due to endorphins.

Finally, imaging experiments could tie brain events and chemical pathways to the person's story or meaning. We might finally be able to trace the complete set of connections between a person's story of the illness, the resulting brain activation, the chemicals released, and the final stages of bodily healing.

While there's a great deal more we want to know about the placebo response and the inner pharmacy, we already know enough to have some reasonable answers, including ways to help ourselves heal better and faster. We have also seen how future research might tell us many more things that we could use to promote healing. Yet, in order for that research to be of the highest quality, it is necessary to be sure it is actually studying the placebo response, not some other natural process which merely resembles it. This leads to the question of what other processes might mimic the placebo response, which we'll explore in the next chapter.

TEN

The Placebo Response and Its Mimics

"If you take three groups, one given no treatment, a second given placebos, and a third given the test drug, you will very often find that the group given the placebos get along very much better, have a much higher percentage of cures than those without treatment, and, perhaps, almost as many as those with the test drug, in some cases more."

—Dr. Eugene F. DuBois, 1946

As we move from theory into practice, I want to readdress a problem we've encountered while studying the placebo response: It is far from the only reason why our bodies might heal. Consequently, there's always a possibility that we'll think the response is operating when in fact another form of healing is at work. If we confuse the real placebo response with other healing factors, how can we be sure that we are getting good advice about taking charge of our own inner pharmacies? It's very much in our interest to have a complete list of all of the mimics of the placebo response.

Let's start off our investigation with a telling case study.

The Hawthorne Effect

In 1927, Elton Mayo, an industrial psychologist, and his associates undertook a major experiment in industrial organization at a branch of the Western Electric Company in Cicero, Illinois. Hoping to demonstrate which changes in the workplace produced the greatest changes in productivity, they systematically altered the wages, hours, rest periods, organization, and amount of supervision of a group of female workers. Although they carefully recorded the results of the various changes, their data were confusing, even contradictory.

Mayo and his team subsequently reanalyzed that data and arrived at a new insight. It appeared that none of the specific alterations they thought they were measuring had any real or lasting effects on workers' behavior. The women did indeed increase their productivity and were generally happier and better adjusted. But, in the last analysis, the improvements seemed to be due solely to the fact that the research team was watching them carefully and recording their activities. As a result of this extra attention, the workers apparently felt more important; hence, their level of performance rose.

Since the experiment was conducted in a factory called the Hawthorne Works, the positive effect of experimental observation alone eventually came to be called "the Hawthorne Effect."

There's another reason why it's worthwhile to study the various factors that might mimic the placebo response, one to which I've alluded before. Such an inquiry will allow us to discuss criticism which you are sure to encounter if you continue reading about placebos: that, contrary to what we have been saying thus far in this book, the placebo response is essentially not a mystery, but a myth.

The Placebo Myth: A Minority Opinion

Of the many thoughtful scientists who have studied and written about the placebo response in the past fifty years, the vast majority have concluded that the phenomenon is real—though they may have disagreed about its precise extent and how to explain its functioning. Still, a small number of critics have argued that the majority has somehow been deluded. It's tempting to ignore this minority opinion, but if we are going to be scientific in our approach, we can't simply dismiss criticism. One determinant of true scientific attitude is pursuing with equal zeal evidence that goes against one's favorite theory as well as evidence that supports it. A central intent of this book is to assess *all* the scientific evidence—both positive and negative—for the placebo response and the inner pharmacy.

Drs. Gunver Kienle and Helmut Kiene, heads of a research institute in Freiburg, Germany, recently published a skeptical analysis of the placebo response. There are two reasons to focus on Kienle-Kiene: They provide an unusually complete list of placebo response mimics and their analysis is the most comprehensive and detailed attempt to debunk the placebo response I have yet encountered. No one can charge that they have been hasty in their judgment, as Kienle and Kiene list 167 references, and claim to have carefully reviewed about a thousand scientific studies in their search for incontrovertible evidence of a placebo response. Our focus will first turn to Kienle and Kiene's analysis of the work of a scientist you've met several times in previous chapters, Dr. Henry Beecher.

The Background: Beecher

We know that Dr. Henry Beecher's 1955 paper, "The Powerful Placebo," got the ball rolling in terms of general acceptance of the placebo response among physicians. Kienle and Kiene start their skeptical assessment by going back to the Beecher paper, and find a lot of reasons for their skepticism.

The Germans feel that Beecher, in retrospect, was much more enthusiastic than careful. Kienle and Kiene found that Beecher made numerous errors in reviewing fifteen other studies—each of which Beecher claimed provided evidence for a strong placebo response. Kienle and Kiene insist that Beecher patently misquoted ten of the fifteen studies and confused a number of mimics with true placebo responses. In sum, Kienle and Kiene claim that if all we had to go on was Beecher's paper and the fifteen studies to which it refers, we'd have absolutely no evidence to conclude that a placebo response exists at all.

The sorts of errors Beecher made were common in the 1940s and 1950s, when modern research methods were in their infancy. Kienle and Kiene proceeded to ask: Have placebo studies gotten to be more reliable in the last couple of decades? Their conclusion is "No."

Let's look now at the various errors Kienle and Kiene allege occur in these more recent papers—all of which mistake one of a number of mimics for a true placebo response.

Natural History and Spontaneous Healing

We saw in our historical review (chapter 2) that even in the nineteenth century, people understood that if you got better after taking a sugar or bread pill, it could be because the disease ran its natural course, unaffected by the mind or the imagination. Whenever you resort to a modern double-blind randomized controlled trial as a source of data on the placebo response, you risk committing the same error, since this type of trial is essentially unconcerned with discerning the difference between a placebo response and the natural history of the illness.

Such a study design can tell us only the difference between the effect caused by the chemical properties of the drug being tested, and everything else. For purposes of the randomized trial, the placebo response and the natural history of the illness are tossed together into the same wastebasket category. For this reason, Kienle and Kiene list natural history as the first important mimic of the placebo response, and cite a study of the common cold which Beecher reviewed in 1955.

The study showed that patients taking placebos were 30 percent improved after six days. Kienle and Kiene assert—quite reasonably, in my view—that this was much more likely to represent the spontaneous healing rate of the illness. Indeed, I'd go them one better and suggest that colds ought to be *more* than 30 percent improved after six days, so perhaps what was seen here was actually a nocebo effect.

Suppose you set out to design the ideal medical experiment for differentiating with certainty between the natural history of the disease and the placebo response. How would you set up your test? You would obviously need more than two groups; a regular-medicine arm and a placebo arm would not do the job. Some experiments have been done with three groups: a regular-medicine arm; a placebo arm; and a no-treatment arm (as Dr. DuBois stated back in 1946). By comparing the placebo arm and the no-treatment arm, you could tell whether any healing resulted from the placebo response or from the natural history of the disease. Some experts have even stated that you should have a fourth arm, in which patients receive the regular drug but don't know they're getting any medicine at all—maybe you snuck it into their morning cup of coffee! Clearly, there are serious ethical problems with conducting an experiment like this, even if it could reveal very pertinent scientific information.

The important point about these more-than-two-armed experiments is that they are much more complicated and difficult to conduct than the common two-armed randomized controlled trial. In addition, they give us little or no extra information about the regular drug. They can only inform us about the natural history of the illness and the placebo response. But the vast majority of research studies are carried out by people primarily concerned about the drug's efficacy. It's unlikely that pharmaceutical companies would pay the extra money and take the extra time to do three- or four-armed experiments. Therefore, in most cases, we will not have direct information about whether a healing effect seen in the placebo arm is a true placebo response or natural history.

Attribution of Symptom Change

All of us have occasional minor symptoms—a twinge of nausea, a fleeting soreness in a muscle—most of which we just ignore. If these symptoms just happen to occur while we are enrolled in a research trial, and someone is asking us to keep a careful record of any drug side effects, then we are likely to report these purely random events as caused by the drug that we are taking—even if what we are really taking is placebo. Kienle and Kiene believe this is where most reports of placebo side effects come from.

Regression to the Mean

This rather forbidding term can be translated into simple English: If you follow a biological measurement which tends to have a natural variation within limits—for example, blood pressure or heart rate—subjects who are currently at the high or low end of the limits will naturally tend to return toward the average "normal" measurement as time passes. Similarly, subjects beginning at the average point are likely to vary upward or downward in the next time period. If you ignore the subjects who are now average, and focus instead on the subjects who are abnormally high or low, then you will get the false idea that "normalization" is happening during the next time period.

To give an example: You select one hundred people whose present blood pressure is 150/95. That, you know, is on the high side of the pressure range. When you measure their blood pressures an hour later, you'll probably find the vast majority will be lower. On the other hand, if you had begun by studying subjects whose pressure was 120/80, then came back in an hour, a certain number of them would most likely have pressures of 150/95. Looking at the entire sample, you'd realize you saw random variation with no predictable pattern at all. But, because initially you'd looked only at the people with abnormally high blood pressure and ignored the subjects displaying normal blood pressure, your data seem to show a trend toward overall improvement.

Suppose that instead of simply measuring blood pressure after the waiting period, you'd given all one hundred of your "hypertensive" group a sugar pill. An hour later, many of them would have dropped to 120/80. Wouldn't you then assume that you'd seen a substantial placebo response? Really, though, what you would have observed was random variation (a species of the natural history of human blood pressure).

Hawthorne and Clinic Effects

As we learned, the Hawthorne effect is the tendency of people to improve in behavior and functioning simply because you are staring at them and recording what they do. Closely related to the Hawthorne effect in medical research is the clinic effect, which refers to the fact that subjects of medical experiments do not *simply* get the "active" drug or the placebo. They also get a good deal of medical attention—because they have to be diagnosed as having all the features needed to participate in the experiment, and their body functions have to be measured regularly. Therefore, they visit clinics more often than most people, and they may get much more thorough physical exams and laboratory tests. Small problems are likely to be picked up sooner and treated more effectively; and having to come back so often may be a strong incentive to take better care of their health. This intensive level of clinical care could cause an improvement in health among the patients taking placebos, and subsequently be misinterpreted as a placebo response.

The Obliging Subject

It's natural for patients to want to please their physicians and for those who volunteer to be subjects in experiments to want to please the investigators. Given these factors, there is a strong psychological tendency for the patient/subject to tell these authority figures what he thinks they want to hear. If a study is designed to measure pain, where the subject's verbal report is the *only* possible measurement, it's especially likely that persons trying to please the investigator will claim that their pain has lessened when perhaps it hasn't. In this situation, the subject's report mimics one in which a true placebo response has occurred.

"Real" Treatment in Placebo Group

Kienle and Kiene believe that in at least some placebo studies, the so-called placebo group actually got a form of active medication, and so any improvement would be due to that medication and not to symbolic meaning or expectancy. It might seem absurd to accuse scientists of making this mistake; how stupid would they have to be to allow the placebo group to get real treatment and not realize it? But in some situations it's very difficult to administer both a placebo and no treatment at the same time.

Consider a double-blind experiment of a topical cream for a skin disease. The placebo cream may not have a certain active chemical. But if it looks and feels enough like a cream to fool the patient, then won't it have at least some soothing properties for the skin? And couldn't any improvement be due to those soothing properties?

With this list, we have reviewed almost all the factors that Kienle and Kiene believe have mimicked true placebo responses, creating the widespread impression that these responses exist. As good scientists seeking to understand the placebo response, we need to be aware that each one is an important source of possible experimental confusion.

How Strong Is the Case Against the Placebo Response?

Drs. Kienle and Kiene's goal was to convince us that *all* reports of the placebo response were due to one of these mimics—that there is no real scientific evidence that the placebo response exists.

The two scientists admit to evidence contrary to their hypothesis. Studies like those of Luparello (remember the asthmatics in chapter 5) persuaded Kienle and Kienle that there *can* be a placebo response in asthma. They immediately limit their admission by asserting that asthma is a unique disease. Asthmatics, they claim, can be made worse by suggestion in a fashion unique to the condition; we shouldn't be surprised that suggestion can also make them better. They caution that we shouldn't extrapolate from this singular case and assume a placebo response exists for any other disease.

Just how plausible is it that there exists precisely one *and only one* disease in which the mind is capable of altering bodily function by means of the placebo response? I suggest that it's not very plausible.

In some sections of their article, Kienle and Kiene do in fact engage in a careful assessment of the scientific data; in other places, though, they make their case simply by adopting a convenient definition. Kienle and Kiene absolutely refuse to call anything a placebo effect unless a placebo—that is, dummy treatment—has been given. That means that almost every bodily change I attribute to the meaning model or to the inner pharmacy Kienle and Kiene would call instead a psychosomatic effect—which, they admit, is extremely powerful. In no way do Kienle and Kiene want to reject or minimize the power of the mind to affect the body. In this way, they could agree with most of what I've written here while still insisting there is no true placebo response.

It's virtually impossible to resolve a definitional dispute of this type. I prefer to think that the placebo response is closely connected with other forms of mind-body healing reactions, which explains my expanded definition. How consistent is it to admit the power of mind-body healing generally, and deny the evidence for the placebo response? Why should the mind exert such a powerful influence over the body in all settings except one—when the influence on the mind comes via the use of a dummy medication or treatment?

The majority opinion on the placebo response relates it to other psychosomatic phenomena. Taking that view, we regard strong evidence for other mind-body responses as indirect evidence of the power of the placebo response, and vice versa. In this case I find the majority view far more plausible than Kienle and Kiene's insistence on putting the placebo response and other forms of mind-body healing in discrete categories.

The type of research that Kienle and Kiene are engaged in is what statisticians would call a meta-analysis: a research study of research studies. Other people actually do the original research, then the authors of the meta-analysis line up a series of research studies side-by-side to see what overall trends can be found when the results are taken as a whole body of research. This is what Dan Moerman did in his review of the thirty-one studies of cimetidine for ulcers, which we read about in chapter 4.

One of the most highly skilled meta-analysis groups currently investigating the placebo response is a team at the University of Amsterdam. Recently, they reviewed all the studies they could find that are more-than-two-armed randomized, clinical placebo-controlled trials. As we saw previously, this is the study design which is best able to separate the placebo response from its most common mimic, the natural history of the illness. The result clearly showed, to the Amsterdam group, that the placebo response exists and can be measured.

For the remainder of this book, I will be advising you on various practices and activities which, in my experience, have been associated with healing. Everything I tell you has solid evidence to back it up. Most of the evidence has already been mentioned in the scientific chapters.

We have talked about both conventional medicine and alternative medicine as two different types of healing practices. What does the placebo response have to do with the relationship between these two approaches to healing? In the next chapter we will examine the placebo response and inner pharmacy as the intersection between these different schools of medicine.

ELEVEN

The Inner Pharmacy at the Interface: Conventional and Alternative Medicine

"The real issue for conventional medicine here is not how to manage our patients' involvement in alternative care; it is rather, in T. S. Eliot's phrase, how to learn from alternative practices in an effort to regain the knowledge we have lost in information."

— Dr. Frank Davidoff, 1998

The placebo response and the inner pharmacy constitute an intersection, or meeting place, between conventional and alternative medicine. This development seems auspicious, because conventional medicine today seems to have a higher level of respect for, and interest in, alternative medicine than at any time since Benjamin Franklin first used that blinded experimental trial to debunk mesmerism.

In comparing these two approaches to healing, it's important to keep in mind that *both* the "conventional" and the "alternative" labels cover an extremely wide range of practices. Often the labels obscure more than they explain. At one extreme within conventional medicine, you might encounter a surgeon who believes that the ideal patient is one who's anesthetized and can't ask annoying questions. At the other extreme are conventional physicians dedicated to the importance of the mind-body connection, who feel it essential that the patient be actively involved in all aspects of care. Similarly, within alternative medicine, some practitioners use an extremely holistic style and devote time to forming relationships with their clients, while others may simply throw a bottle of herbal tablets at you and say, "Take these." It's one thing to make generalizations about these large classes of treatments and practices, and quite a different thing to assess carefully any one alternative (or conventional) practitioner or treatment.

Therapy That Fits

An anthropologist studying a group of chiropractors and their patients set out to discover why the chiropractors enjoyed such a high level of patient loyalty. He noted that the chiropractors and their patients tended to come from working-class backgrounds, unlike most of the conventional physicians with practices in the same part of town. He also observed that the patients were comfortable viewing the world in terms of machinery, and that the chiropractors were much more likely than conventional physicians to use mechanical images when explaining a condition to a patient.

This had a "double positive" effect: It provided an explanation which made good sense to the patients; and it demonstrated that the chiropractors were their kind of people. The chiropractors were able to cement a stronger relational bond than conventional physicians.

Any responsible physician would find it difficult to ignore such telling data. Yet we know all too well the long history of hostility between what we today call conventional medicine and other schools of healing. As recently as the 1950s and 1960s, the American Medical Association launched a relentless public relations campaign against chiropractors, stopping its barrage only when forced to do so by a federal antitrust injunction. That hostility seems to be sharply in decline today.

Conventional Medicine Looks at Alternative Medicine

Why does conventional medicine seem to be taking a more sympathetic view of alternative medicine? For one thing, American physicians are members of American society. If society as a whole finds alternative medicine as fascinating and attractive as it appears to, eventually physicians cannot help being influenced as well. It's no longer unusual to find conventional M.D.'s who have studied one or more alternative styles of healing, even incorporating them into their practices for selected patients.

The movement in American medicine to acknowledge patient rights and patient freedom to choose has likewise had an impact on the legitimization of alternative techniques. If the patient elects to consult with alternative healers, then the conventional physician has two choices: to remain blind to this fact; or to talk frankly with the patient, become informed about the alternative treatment, and determine how the conventional and alternative treatments could best work together.

If the physician chooses the latter course, he will end up considerably better informed about alternative medicine. Once this communication has occurred, it will become much more difficult to maintain an attitude of general distrust and scorn toward alternative medicine, especially when he's witnessing its apparent successes.

Finally, conventional physicians have always prided themselves on their scientific achievements, curiosity, skills, and research. It had to dawn on them eventually that ignoring alternative medicine—and refusing even to consider researching its methods and results—was simply unscientific.

It was popular pressure on Congress, rather than the demands of the scientific medical community, that created an Office of Alternative Medicine at the National Institutes of Health. This office, now upgraded to a center, has further legitimized research into alternative medicine and has assured that at least some money, though much less than for conventional research, would be devoted to this purpose: seeking ways to encourage clinical interaction between both schools of treatment.

In fact, Dr. Andrew Weil, always a prominent advocate of alternative treatment regimens, has suggested that the wave of the future is going to be what he calls integrative medicine—conventional and alternative medicine employed side-by-side by practitioners who respect, teach, and communicate with each other. This, he believes, will finally allow us to discover what works and what doesn't work for the individual condition and patient—insuring that no patient be denied an effective remedy simply because he happens to consult one school of medicine rather than another. The appeal of Dr. Weil's open-minded approach is evidenced by the growing number of conventional physicians applying to study in his program at the University of Arizona.

How does this new open-mindedness affect the reputation and efficacy of the placebo response and the inner pharmacy?

The Placebo Response's Place in Both Alternative and Conventional Medicine

Due to the cross-fertilization between conventional and alternative medicine, the placebo response can at last assume its rightful place at the interface. Remember, both types of healing inevitably have a symbolic impact, affecting the meaning that the patient ascribes to being sick and being healthy. We've seen that changed meaning can turn on the body's inner pharmacy and promote faster healing. If both schools of practitioners can accept this symbolic dimension, they will use it to heal.

Let's proceed with a placebo-response inventory of the two different sorts of healing. One particular generalization about the difference between conventional and alternative medicine is a good place to start: Many types of alternative medicine today probably rely relatively more on the placebo response to get results than do most types of conventional medicine.

At first blush, this may sound as if I'm dismissing alternative medicine. But seeing it this way would fall into the trap I warned of previously—being swayed by the old negative connotation of placebo response instead of seeing it as a positive healing tool. Instead, I simply mean to point out an important fact: Conventional medicine has worked harder than alternative medicine, over recent years, to eliminate treatments which rely largely on the placebo effect to get results. That amounts to saying that conventional medicine has accepted as gospel the results of double-blind randomized controlled trials (RCTs), and that, by definition, if an RCT shows that something works only as well as placebos work, then the treatment is deemed a failure.

Ironically, this mindset has resulted in conventional medicine's ceding a certain part of its turf to alternative medicine. Some diseases cannot be cured by conventional means, and the way conventional medicine tries to manage these conditions may leave much to be desired in the individual's quality of life. Patients often seek alternative medicine for chronic pain and arthritis, precisely because conventional medicine seems able to do little for them.

Alternative medicine has either not been especially interested in carrying out RCTs, or else simply lacked the resources, financial and otherwise, to do them—although this is rapidly changing. This means that treatments which rely strongly upon a placebo response have not been eliminated from alternative medicine.

When you hear reports of patients who feel frustrated in numerous encounters with conventional physicians, but who then feel much more emotionally supported and better understood when they seek the help of alternative healers, you begin to wonder whether alternative medicine, in addition to whatever other benefit it may provide, could be an unusually effective means of releasing a placebo response in patients who are resistant to placebo stimuli within conventional medicine. Some patients may never fully develop their inner pharmacies as long as they see only conventional physicians, but their pharmacies may respond considerably better to the messages sent in by alternative healing modes and practitioners.

The meaning model gives us an especially useful framework for understanding exactly what features of alternative medicine may make it an unusually powerful trigger for the inner pharmacy.

Alternative Medicine, the Meaning Model, and the Inner Pharmacy

The meaning model states that a positive placebo response is most likely to occur when the patient tells his story to an interested listener, gets a satisfying explanation of what is happening and what to do about it, feels cared for and concerned about by the caregiver, and achieves a stronger sense of control over the illness or symptom.

Certain practices within alternative medicine tend to make it highly suited to provide these three elements. In fact, it seems to be so effective that critics within conventional medicine have suggested that their fellow physicians could learn a few lessons from their alternative counterparts.

The first of the three healing conditions listed is explanations. As we've seen, different people prefer different types of explanations for what ails them. Some view themselves as scientifically minded and favor conventional medicine, regarding all alternative theory as mumbo-jumbo. Others consider alternative teachings to be commonsensical. They feel that conventional medicine overwhelms them with a lot of jargon, which allows the conventional physician to retain power and prevents the patient from taking charge.

At least for some people, alternative explanations will make more sense and become more meaningful as ways of dealing with illness. Moreover, those who initially favor conventional approaches, but who do not get better, will eventually seek a different explanation, which may be meaningful to them simply because it holds out new hope.

In a very thoughtful paper, Drs. Ted Kaptchuk and David Eisenberg of Harvard Medical School describe some of the beliefs common to most forms of alternative medicine—beliefs that make such medicine an attractive explanation for many people today:

- Nature and the natural are viewed as wholesome and virtuous. What is natural is good for us. The forces of nature all seem to be lined up on our side.

- There are frequent references to concepts such as "life forces" and "energy." Conventional medical science rejected "vitalism," the belief in a special life force unique to plants and animals, in the mid-nineteenth century, claiming we would only have complete knowledge of living systems when we could fully explain them according to the same physical and chemical laws that apply to nonliving matter. In so doing, conventional medicine deprived itself of a metaphor that to many people is comforting and meaningful.

- Alternative medicine is full of science, only it is a different science from that recognized by conventional physicians. You can, after all, read entire books about alternative medicine and its treatments and spend years learning some of its systems. It's been suggested that the sciences of alternative medicine resemble modern geology and paleontology—which describe the world as it is without trying to do experiments in the laboratory—rather than physics and chemistry — which are favored as the models of good science by medical investigators.

- The spiritual dimension is incorporated into many alternative theories and practices, and today our society seems anxious to recapture a connection with the spiritual. For example, even the daily work of staying healthy can resemble religious ritual; consider, for instance, the practice of brewing herbal teas to maintain well-being or ward off illness. Over time, such simple daily acts can become infused with the meaning of redemption, or of the triumph of the spirit over bodily imperfection. Here's an example which is literally close to home.

Daralyn's Chicken Soup

When our children were small, Daralyn resorted to the traditional remedy of homemade chicken soup to combat colds. As our son Mark got older, he continued to request chicken soup when ill, and asked specifically that Mom make it herself. On one level, this would argue for a conditioned healing response. On another, it would suggest parent and child becoming bonded through a meaningful ritual.

Now let's explore alternative medicine's use of another aspect of our meaning model: caring. Touch is one of the most basic and primitive expressions of caring; that's how we felt cared for when we were babies. Conventional medicine tends to use touch in a very limited way, and in many instances the touching, when it occurs, is painful. Certain types of alternative practices—chiropractic and therapeutic massage, for example—rely heavily on touch and make it a central portion of the treatment. The caring message could come across much more strongly in those treatments.

Alternative healers may also be less rushed and take more time with each patient. Consider homeopathy, which, unlike most other types of alternative medicine, has conducted its own RCTs and concluded that some of its methods are superior to placebo in those studies. That conclusion does not mean that homeopathy has eliminated the placebo response from its arsenal.

A typical homeopathic treatment session relies upon a very detailed history of the patient's symptoms, which may involve discussing a single symptom for up to half an hour. After the visit, a patient will very likely think, "No regular physician has ever spent this much time talking just about my headaches (or my asthma or my backaches or my allergies). This homeopath must really care about me; and the treatment he selected must have been chosen especially with me in mind." Given such a healing environment, the inner pharmacy can hardly avoid lending a helping hand in the healing process.

Next we turn to the control facet of the meaning model. Alternative treatments vary along a spectrum. At one end of that spectrum, the patient being worked on by the practitioner is as passive as he would be in any form of conventional medicine—for example, acupuncture or acupressure. But many alternative treatments, such as those that rely heavily on nutrition and other lifestyle changes, as well as meditation and guided imagery, offer a greater degree of control or participation.

For many patients, this is one of alternative medicine's outstanding attractions. Even when alternative treatments are "done to" you, the sense of control can be greater than in conventional medicine.

Our world is designed to encourage us toward conventional medicine and away from alternative medicine. Most people must to some degree swim against the tide and exercise a bit more control over their own destinies in order to use alternative medicine in the first place. Such persons must search out an alternative practitioner, choose among a bewildering array of treatment methods, and often pay out of pocket. They feel more in control because they did not simply "follow the crowd" to the nearest conventional clinic or hospital.

What about those who do not have to swim against the tide, and who encounter alternative medicine in the daily course of living? These are often people for whom the alternative medical practice is the existing folk or popular medical system of their particular culture or community. A Latina woman living in a Hispanic neighborhood may automatically seek out the local *curandera* before visiting a conventional physician. By doing so, she probably feels more in control of her life: The curandera is a well-known person who respects the same cultural beliefs and practices the woman does; by contrast, the conventional physician may not speak Spanish and may be unfamiliar with aspects of her daily life. He may seem to be a more threatening figure, because—to many people from ethnic subcultures who live in the U.S.—going to the physician and especially to the hospital involves giving up control, forgoing the close support of family and friends, and entering a world of the "unnatural."

The Natural Factor in Healing

Drs. Kaptchuk and Eisenberg observed that many people prefer alternative medicine explicitly because they view it as more natural than conventional medicine. Yet just what is meant by "natural" turns out to be rather difficult to define. One dimension of "natural" is that the treatment strikes us as comfortable and familiar. The treatment's impact upon the body, we believe, is as close as possible to the sorts of processes the body, left to its own devices, carries on by itself. A natural treatment is "gentle," while a different sort of treatment is "harsh." This seems to underscore the point that the more natural we view the treatment as being, the more we are likely to feel in control as it is being administered; the less natural we think the treatment is, the more we are likely to feel that we have given up control of ourselves and of our bodies.

To the skeptic or critic of alternative medicine, this way of thinking seems completely illogical. As I have mentioned, such critics enjoy pointing out that such poisons as hemlock and arsenic are naturally occurring substances, and that the chemical structure of vitamins manufactured in a laboratory is identical to that of naturally occurring vitamins. These critics err by not engaging in the discussion at the level that matters most to the patient: the symbolic level. At the symbolic level, there is a logical connection between the idea of natural and the idea of being in control. Alternative medicine may, at the symbolic level, create a sense of control in a general, indirect way. At a practical level, such therapies may lead to enhanced self-control since they are directed at lifestyle changes or other measures a person can take on his own.

Imagine a cancer patient who has been treated first by surgery, then by chemotherapy. Now she is using herbal and nutritional remedies to build up her strength and to prevent the cancer from recurring. She takes certain pills or capsules at certain times of the day and restricts her diet to specific foods. This person has basically taken complete control over the course of her treatment. Perhaps no alternative practitioner was consulted at all. She might have discovered this program of herbal and nutritional support from a book or on the Internet. In this regard, taking care of your own body is very much a do-it-yourself project.

The use of the alternative approach makes the patient once again feel directly in control. In this case, the cancer itself becomes less of a threat simply because it is open to being managed by relatively simple, natural means.

If the only means to eliminate cancer is to cut my body open with knives and to bombard my bloodstream with poisonous chemicals, then cancer is terrifying and out of my control—requiring that I surrender my body to powerful outside forces. Once I decide I can keep the cancer out of my body by natural means, I greatly reduce the threat posed by disease and immediately feel much more in control of my own destiny. The cancer now *means* something very different to me than it did before. This, in turn, increases the chance that I'll turn on whatever cancer-fighting substances can be found in my inner pharmacy.

Using Alternative Medicine Logically

One of the first large studies to try to discover how people use alternative medicine was carried out by Dr. David Eisenberg and his colleagues at Harvard Medical School, and published in 1993. Eisenberg's team surveyed a random sample of adults across the U.S. and found that 34 percent had used some form of alternative medicine in the previous year. Indeed, they calculated that Americans made more visits to alternative practitioners than they did to primary care M.D.'s (family physicians, general internists, and general pediatricians) during the same time period.

Dr. Eisenberg also calculated the out-of-pocket sums that Americans paid for alternative medicine equaled the out-of-pocket money paid for all forms of conventional medicine. To say the least, this was an eye-opening study for many conventional physicians, who previously had no idea that alternative medicine was so widespread. It also encouraged many HMOs and medical centers to become interested in alternative medicine, just to get a piece of the money people are willing to spend.

Dr. Eisenberg's study didn't do much to reveal the thoughts of those who chose to use alternative medicine. Dr. John Astin, of Stanford Medical School, set out to do a national study which would better answer those questions.

Using a written survey, Dr. Astin found out that about 40 percent of his sample had used some form of alternative medicine, the most popular being chiropractic, lifestyle and diet, exercise and movement, and relaxation techniques. The most common conditions for which people used these alternative methods were anxiety, chronic fatigue, muscle strains, arthritis, and headaches.

According to the answers Astin received, you were more likely to use alternative medicine if you:

- Were better educated.
- Were excited by personal growth psychology and liked to try new things.
- Had previously had a transformative experience that changed your worldview.
- Felt your overall health was poorer than it should be.
- Possessed a holistic health philosophy (believing in the importance of mind, body, and spirit).
- Had such specific health problems as anxiety, chronic pain, and back problems, which seemed to resist conventional treatment.

As you can see from this list, the best answer to Dr. Astin's basic question was that people chose alternative medicine because it was a better fit with their philosophy of life and health than for any other reason. Dissatisfaction with conventional medicine and a desire to stay in control did *not* correlate strongly with use of alternative practices. In fact, the vast majority of people queried used alternative medicine in addition to conventional medicine, not instead of it.

What can we learn from Astin's study? Two points stand out. First, people tend to use what seems to work for them. If conventional medicine solves their problems, they will use conventional medicine. The problems that most people take to alternative medicine are precisely those for which conventional medicine tends to have the least successful track record. In this way, most people's use of alternative medicine seems wise and logical—the very opposite of behaving as if they were brainwashed or hoodwinked into seeking something weird or unusual, which is the attitude of groups like "Quackwatch," one of the most commonly recommended web sites for "accurate, scientific" information about alternative practices.

Dr. Astin's findings also help reassure conventional practitioners about one of their worst fears: that patients with diseases easily treatable by conventional medicine will delay the correct diagnosis for a long time because of their devotion to alternative medicine, so that by the time they get to a regular physician, it will be too late to cure the disease.

Dr. Astin's point that people want their health care to dovetail with their values and beliefs again paints a picture of a very logical and thoughtful choice of healing practice. "Different strokes for different folks" may explain what most effectively activates our inner pharmacies.

Alternative and Conventional Medicine: The Interface

In order to explain why alternative medicine might be an especially powerful way to stimulate the inner pharmacy, I have portrayed conventional medicine in a rather stark and uncompromising way, stressing that it puts the RCT on a pedestal as the only legitimate way of knowing anything about disease and its treatment. I must now add that the same defects, which the public at large and alternative healers see in conventional medicine, are increasingly appreciated by its own practitioners. Many of the things we've discussed in this chapter as ways that alternative medicine can best stimulate the inner pharmacy are being taught widely in medical schools as the most humanistic and compassionate way for the modern physician to help the patient.

Spending more time talking with the patient; focusing upon the creation of positive relationships; using touch appropriately as part of the average medical visit; attending to the patient's spiritual as well as physical and mental concerns—all these issues are getting more and more attention in the training of tomorrow's conventional physicians. I would seriously mislead you if I caused you to think that only in an alternative practitioner could you find these ideal healing qualities.

If the forward-looking educators of tomorrow's physicians are right, then the aspects of alternative medicine we have been focusing upon in this chapter will provide a model for all of medical practice, not only alternative medicine. This model of medical practice smoothly integrates the placebo response into the basic, everyday pattern of caring for patients—and, in doing so, hands a lot of control back to the patients. The practitioner of either type of medicine can then approach each patient visit with the question, "What can I do to assist your inner pharmacy in contributing to the healing process?"

Helping to turn on the patient's own inner healing processes is a noble goal. But remember the old saying: "Give a man a fish and you feed him for a day; teach him to fish and you feed him for a lifetime." If we have learned anything at all in the past eleven chapters, it is that there are many ways of stimulating a placebo response, and no special skill or training seems necessary for many of them. After all, if Mom could do it by putting Band-Aids on our bumps and scrapes or by making chicken soup, why can't we follow in her footsteps?

We've now arrived at the point of using what we've learned about the science of the placebo response to empower us to trigger the inner pharmacy to assist in our own healing. We'll start, in the next chapter, with some factors that can either aid or interfere with self-healing and discover how to encourage or overcome them.

TWELVE

Clearing a Path for the Inner Pharmacy: Desire and Forgiveness

"And to the degree that I can . . . have . . . compassion for my own ignorance and my own darkness and my own inner demons, then I can begin to have that same compassion and love for other people whenever they display their darkness to me. When I can do that, it helps to free us both."

—Dr. Dean Ornish

"You have to want to get better." At first, this piece of advice seems so obvious as to be almost insulting. Doesn't everyone who is ill desire wellness? Wouldn't anybody prefer health to sickness? As it turns out, that's not necessarily true. And, in any case, just how does desire affect healing?

Desire: Its Critical Role in Our Health

I've already cited early placebo studies that implicate desire to improve in an indirect way. While studying the response of wounded soldiers in World War II, Dr. Henry Beecher noticed important differences in how much and what type of pain they seemed to feel. Given our present context, we may wonder about the extent to which soldiers wanted to get better as their wounds were being treated.

Getting better would—as we mentioned earlier—almost certainly mean returning to the front lines and having to face death once again. In those circumstances, just how potent a desire to heal would a normal human being display? On a conscious level, of course, these soldiers were loyal and patriotic and were eager to go on serving their country. But could you blame them if, at a subconscious level, their desire to heal was really quite low? Knowing what we do now about the inner pharmacy, we can readily imagine that a subconscious lack of desire could directly affect the rate of improvement in bodily health.

More recently, as we saw in chapter 5, Drs. Donald Price and Howard Fields have reviewed the experimental data on placebo pain relief and have argued that in order to predict how a placebo will work, you must know two things about the subjects: whether they expect to improve and whether they desire to improve.

Expectancy and Desire

A great number of studies have looked at expectations; but very few have examined desire, perhaps because the investigators simply assumed that everyone desires to improve if he has pain. Yet the few studies which have been done confirm that the response to placebo varies with differing levels of desire; and that if you can mathematically combine the expectancy score and the desire score, you will have a better predictor of placebo response than if you looked at either score alone.

Here's a striking case of how lack of desire to improve can block *both* the inner and the outer pharmacies.

Fighting Against the Medicine

This anecdote was told at a conference on the placebo response by Dr. Godehard Oepen, a psychiatrist at the Bedford, Massachusetts VA Hospital responsible for a schizophrenic patient whom we will call "Rodney." Rodney was about twenty-five years old and had been hospitalized by court order for his severe and violent psychotic symptoms. When Dr. Oepen tried to talk with Rodney, he angrily refused to communicate with the psychiatrist.

The treatment prescribed for Rodney was the antipsychotic drug haloperidol, which ought to have controlled most of his symptoms, or at least made him groggy and dopey. Surprisingly, the drug seemed to have almost no effect, even though the nurses could testify he was getting the complete series of injections.

Every day Dr. Oepen would go to see Rodney and patiently attempt to explain why the treatment could help him, or at least try to find out why he was rejecting help. And every day Rodney cursed him and refused to interact. This went on for five or six weeks, with the medication failing to produce any improvement despite increases in dosage.

Then two surprising events occurred. First, Rodney began to talk with Dr. Oepen. He told him, "You know, doctor, you've been seeing me every day and have always been polite. You never got angry even though I've been horrible to you. So I was thinking—why don't I give this a chance and do it your way? I'll just take pills—you don't have to give me injections."

The second occurence was that Rodney became extremely sedated by the haloperidol. Overnight, he went from being hostile and combative to almost comatose—even though he was off the injections and taking the medication orally. At this point, he was getting a huge dose of the drug, and the staff had to cut the dose way back. Rodney also began to display a Parkinson's-like tremor in his hands, a common side effect of major tranquilizers like haloperidol, especially when they are given at high doses for long periods, but Rodney had shown no tremors in the previous five to six weeks he'd been taking it.

"You know, I was fighting that drug the entire time you were injecting it," Rodney later told Dr. Oepen. "I was really hating you and the system and everything. I could feel the drug effect coming on and I was fighting it off, but it was hard. When I agreed to the pills, though, I just let it take over, just let myself give in." From that moment on, Rodney made a dramatic improvement with the haloperidol: He got markedly better within a week, while most patients starting out on the drug require a longer time for full benefit.

Rodney's case is an unusual but instructive one. Fortunately, few patients have such extreme opposition to the desire to get better. Since Rodney's insights into his own state of mind correlate so well with the outward signs that Dr. Oepen observed, this case study may give us a clue about the workings of the inner pharmacy. For six weeks, it was almost as if Rodney was calling a prescription to his own inner pharmacy, and the prescription was for *the antidote to haloperidol.*

In chapter 9, we saw that the drug naloxone is a very potent blocker of morphine, as well as of endorphins. Give a person a huge overdose of morphine, then five minutes later give that same person a shot of naloxone, and almost instantly it will appear as if that person had been given no morphine at all. Rodney seemed to have the capability of phoning up his own inner pharmacy and administering himself doses of whatever natural blocker works like naloxone for haloperidol. As soon as he stopped calling in those prescriptions to his inner pharmacy, the drug he was taking was freed to function.

Rodney's story makes us consider the possibility that an even milder lack of desire to get better can retard our inner pharmacy, rather than promote healing. If you want to make sure that your inner pharmacy is doing all it can to help improve your condition, you must want to improve as much as possible. In saying this, we must beware of the pitfall of thinking of the mind-body relationship as if it were a recipe with 100 percent positive results.

Avoiding the Pitfall of "Judge-and-Blame"

The pitfall I call the "judge and blame" approach adds tremendously to the misery caused by diseases like cancer. It's the assumption that patients who get worse and who die must have failed, and must themselves have caused their own deterioration, because they obviously didn't want to get better. I emphatically reject this mind-set every bit as strongly as I accept the validity of mind-body medicine. I'm not talking here about people who get sicker because of negative lifestyle choices like smoking, but rather about cases where a "lack of desire" seems to be the *only* explanation for a patient's treatment failure.

The advice I am offering in this book is forward-looking: You presently have a health problem or issue, and you want to increase the odds you'll get better or keep the condition under control longer. Right now, I cannot predict with certainty how well things are going to work out for you. My approach is quite different from backward-looking judgments, which start from knowing how things went—for instance, that your condition deteriorated—and then try to assign blame by insisting you must not have *really* tried hard enough.

Judging and blaming, the ultimate backward look, seem seriously misguided for two reasons. First, it can be self-serving. The blamer is frequently an advocate or practitioner of a mind-body healing technique. Rather than admit that the technique may not be perfect, he attacks the victim to make himself look and feel superior—or even, in a worst case scenario, to bring in more business.

The blamer may also be suffering from the same disease as the person being blamed. This blamer is terrified of dying and has a deep psychological need to put as much distance as possible between himself and any "treatment failures." Most of us tend to do this unconsciously—when, for example, we hear that someone our own age has died. "*I'm* not going to die," is my reaction. "*I* work out at the gym five times a week." A good way to establish this distance is for the scared person to say, "*I* really want to get better and *I* am really trying; that other person was always thinking negative thoughts and must have brought it on himself." This may make the blamer feel better momentarily, but it's relief purchased at the price of unrealistic thinking and a serious lack of compassion and understanding.

The second, more deep-seated reason I reject "judge and blame" is that the body's response to most diseases like cancer is complex. My cancer may be a slowly growing and nonaggressive sort of cell, or it may be a highly malignant cell type. The cancer cells may be exquisitely sensitive to radiation or chemotherapy treatments; or they may be highly resistant. My own body defenses may be strong, or other diseases from which I suffer may have weakened them. I may come from a hardy family, or one in which many members have died early from similar cancers.

All of these factors combine with the mind-body healing forces to determine the outcome of my struggle against the disease. To claim that how much I want to get better is the only determinant of the outcome grossly oversimplifies the actual situation.

Many of the factors listed above are simply beyond our control. It makes good sense, in our efforts to help ourselves, to focus especially on those aspects of illness we can control. When we adopt the forward-looking posture, we can emphasize our desire to recover from illness, but let's do this with both humility and empathy. When someone's life has already been cursed by the spread or regrowth of cancer or some other serious illness, let's not add to his unhappiness by suggesting that he brought it on himself—especially when such a claim has no scientific support.

Keeping in mind our goal of avoiding blame, let's now return to our initial question: Doesn't anyone, automatically, desire to get better when ill; and so can't we assume that this desire is already at its highest pitch?

Lack of Desire to Improve

The goal of this part of the book is self-help, not making judgments about other people; so let's be bold and tough self-critics. If we are, we may find that our desire to get better is interconnected with other psychological urges which could block an optimal placebo response. This awareness could enable us to connect to our inner pharmacies more effectively.

It's normal for people who live with chronic disease for a sustained time period to organize portions of their lives around the illness. This can be a completely healthy adaptation—for instance, a diabetic's familiarizing herself with the required diet and exercising on a regular basis to shed excess pounds. When we begin to organize our lives in such a manner, we become in one way or another defined by our disease. Our disease becomes part of our identity. Finally, it may just be too frightening to surrender such a defining part of ourselves.

Caroline Myss, in her popular book *Why People Don't Heal and How They Can,* has summarized very well how this happens:

> ***"I believe that many of us are almost as afraid of healing as we are of illness. . . . Illness can, for instance, be a powerful way to get attention you might not otherwise receive—as a form of leverage, illness can seem almost attractive. Illness may also convey the message that you have to change your life quite drastically. Because change is among the most frightening aspects of life, you may fear change more intensely than illness and enter into a pattern of postponing the changes you need to make."***

For people with low self-esteem, Myss concludes, feelings of guilt, a sense of failure, even of shame can be justified or explained away by the advent of illness—after all, a sick person cannot be expected to function well in the world. She reminds us that these rationalized feelings can extend beyond self-flagellation for perceived failures; they may affect our deepest sense of relationships with others.

For some psychologically wounded people, becoming healthy and attaining independence amounts to isolation and vulnerability. For many, this fear of heroic independence—and by extension, of being alone—lies at the core of their inability to heal. Here's an example cited by Myss.

Clinging to Illness

Meg, a woman in her fifties, had suffered from back and leg pain for many years and failed to respond to various attempts at treatment. To make matters worse, a relationship she'd hoped would lead to marriage had recently ended; apparently the boyfriend had been looking for a wealthier wife. Still, her ex-beau continued to visit Meg daily since the pain limited her mobility, and she had no one else to help her with her daily activities.

> ***"I then asked her if she thought that becoming healthy meant that this man would no longer have a reason to visit her. Meg's***

response was so rapid that I don't think she realized what she said. 'I can't get healthy. He would leave me and find someone else, and then what would I do?'"

I interpret Myss as saying it's very unlikely that Meg's inner pharmacy will come to her assistance to deal with the pain in her back and legs. I would add that Meg's inner pharmacy seems to be receiving two conflicting messages. The surface message is that she wants to be free of the pain and able to do things that the pain now prevents. The deeper, subconscious message—which for Meg is the more real expression of her mind—says that the pain is a critically important piece of herself. Without it, she'd be alone and helpless. So the inner pharmacy is going to listen to the deeper, real message and avoid doing anything that could diminish the pain.

Now, let's see what you can do on your own to help determine whether any such subconscious messages may be standing in your way of your healing.

A Desire Inventory

Admittedly, many if not most people who feel like Meg are in denial. Telling them to wake up to what they're really feeling isn't going to work. There are, however, some questions you can ask yourself which will provide useful clues to the message you're actually sending to your inner pharmacy. Remember, you're going to be a tough self-critic.

1. Did you grow up being told, in one way or another, that you were not a very good person? Regardless of whether that has made you adopt some hidden desire to stay ill, you might feel much better, and function much better, if you considered counseling for this problem.
2. Ask yourself the question: "What would my life be like if this health problem (my migraine headaches, my back pain, or whatever) suddenly and completely disappeared?" The "right" answer to this question, we have been trained to think, is, "Well, for joy, for joy, wouldn't my life then be completely grand." And so this is

the answer we are likely to think of when we ask the question.

If we pay extremely close attention to our inner voices, we might be alert to a momentary hesitation before the "right" answer pops out. In that moment of hesitation we might be vaguely conscious of some doubt, some fear, or some anxiety. (Not many of us can be as honest as Meg and blurt out the truth in so many words.) This hesitation may be the best available clue that our desires to become healthy are not pure but are mixed in with some desire or need to cling to our illness. Perhaps, if we focused upon that momentary feeling, we could "see the light"—on our own or, if necessary, with the help of a therapist.

3. If the question we just asked, the very general "what if" question, does not yield any results, it may be that we need to ask more focused ones:

    a) "What role does my illness play, if any, in the degree of responsibility I take for what I do and how I perform?"

    b) "What role does my illness play, if any, in how I relate to my close family and friends, and how they relate to me?"

After posing those questions to yourself and thinking very carefully and deeply about your responses, ask the big "what if it all went away" question again. You might find that if you're honest with yourself, a part of the answer will be, "Then I would really have to finish that project I've successfully been putting off for five years." Or: "Then my family would ignore me and I'd feel lonely." Such answers are tip-offs as to what feelings are really motivating you.

By going through this inventory, you may be enabled to identify some possible sources of your conflicting desires for health and illness. Next, you need to assess whether these conflicts are minor and natural. Feeling ambivalent about such things is probably a basic mark of being human. Perhaps your ambivalence has become serious enough to warrant counseling. A practitioner or healer who's a good listener and communicator is an excellent person to talk to first, especially if you've pinpointed this negative stage and aren't sure how to change it.

If your discussion with the practitioner reveals that ambivalent desires could indeed be putting major roadblocks in the healing path, he may be able to steer you to the right psychologist or other counselor for your problem. It's my experience that these are the sorts of issues that are very hard to resolve completely on our own.

As you start the counseling process, you can have confidence that you are truly doing healing work. By having upbeat and optimistic expectations about what the counseling will do for your health, you're raising the odds that the counseling will succeed.

Our discussion of desire has provided us with further clues as to how our thinking processes (even subconscious ones) may affect the workings of the inner pharmacy. Let's turn now to another mode of thinking which can have a strong impact on our health: forgiveness.

Forgiveness and the Inner Pharmacy

Forgiveness may not at first seem very closely related to the desire to get better, but we have just seen how a hidden desire to remain ill might send exactly the wrong message to the inner pharmacy. Another emotion that can send the wrong message is lack of forgiveness.

From Hate to Healing in Oklahoma City

In the fall of 1998, Bud Welch explained in a newspaper interview how he went from being the father of a bomb victim to an outspoken opponent of the death penalty for the convicted bomber.

Bud's twenty-three-year-old daughter, Julie Marie, was working as a Spanish translator for the Social Security Administration in the Alfred P. Murrah Federal Building in Oklahoma City on April 19, 1995, and became one of the 168 fatalities in the bomb blast for which Timothy McVeigh was later found guilty.

Bud Welch, third of eight children, who had run a service station for more than thirty years, was a high school graduate, a Catholic and a staunch opponent of the death penalty—or so he thought. That comfortable, intellectual view was shattered by his adored daughter's death.

Now, all he could say about the bombers was, "Fry 'em." In his rage, he couldn't see any reason why there should even be a trial. As his fury built month after month, and Timothy McVeigh and Terry Nichols were charged with the bombing, Bud's health began to deteriorate. He was smoking three packs of cigarettes a day and drinking heavily.

Finally, one cold day in January, he went to stand under an old American elm tree, the only object close to the Murrah Building that had survived the blast. Julie, he knew, had liked to park her car under the tree on hot days.

"I started thinking about how miserable I was," he explained later. "I wanted to know how I would be helped after [the bombing suspects] were tried and executed. I struggled with that question for two or three weeks. And I finally realized, it ain't going to help at all. It sure won't bring Julie Marie back. Revenge, hatred, and rage—that's why Julie Marie is dead today."

Bud later saw Timothy McVeigh's father, Bill, on television. "He was this plain, unassuming man like myself. But I saw the pain. Maybe it wasn't visible to others, but it was to me." Eventually Bud arranged to meet Bill McVeigh and found a man who was as destroyed by what had happened to his son as Bud was over the loss of his daughter. After that meeting, Bud was a changed man. He took to public speaking—a role he had always shied away from—to call for clemency for McVeigh's death sentence. "I've somehow felt closer to God than I ever have since I met with Bill," he says. "It was the most satisfying thing I've done in my life. It brought me so much peace, I can't tell you."

Now let's look specifically at the health-related aspects of Bud's story. The old Bud's health was going straight downhill. Besides the smoking and drinking, it's easy to guess that his blood pressure was high and that, if he hadn't actually developed an ulcer, he was certainly at a much higher risk for one. Hearing his story, we wouldn't be surprised if he'd had a heart attack, since he showed all the signs that his stress pathway was in high gear.

By contrast, the new Bud, is likely to be much healthier. Some of his improved health is doubtlessly due to stopping smoking and drinking less, but at least a part of it has to be attributed to the fact that his biochemical pathways are set on health rather than self-destruction mode. I'd call the process Bud went through, a genuine spiritual opening up, forgiveness.

One growing area of modern health research is the link between health and spiritual activities; scientists are finding that prayer and religious dedication can actually make a difference in one's state of health. I firmly believe that research over the next few decades will show us many links between the workings of an individual's inner pharmacy and spiritual life. For now, I will concentrate solely on forgiveness as a way to assure that your inner pharmacy is fully able to hear the healing messages you want to send it. Let's investigate what happens to you when you won't forgive.

Lack of Forgiveness and Your Health

Most people live their daily lives carrying around a load of resentment or even hatred toward others who have done bad things to them in the past. When asked, we always have the very best of reasons for feeling as we do. We can demonstrate that we were blameless and that the other person was completely at fault. Our standard reaction is, "How can you expect me to forgive a person who did a thing like *that*?"

For many of us, this resentment is a pretty minor part of our lives and the anger far from all-consuming. I'll leave it to our spiritual advisers to tell us how important it is for us to address this level of lack of forgiveness. Since my own concern is health-related, I became interested in cases like Bud's, in which a stratospheric level of rage threatens to cause an actual worsening of health, or is interfering in a serious way with getting better from a disease or illness.

In these cases, I believe that the standard answer we give is the wrong way around. We talk about forgiveness—or rather our unwillingness to forgive—as if it all had to do with the *other person.* To forgive, we think, would somehow be to deny how seriously evil or vicious that other person's behavior was. We like to say that doing wrong should have consequences, and it seems to us that forgiving is letting that person off the hook—which would be a denial of our whole system of moral rules. And this may be true, so far as it goes.

What we fail to add to the equation is that forgiveness is not mainly about the other person; rather, it's about *us.* The health-related question is whether we realize the burden or weight we are carrying around with us every day as a result of our accumulated and carefully nurtured rage and anger. Bud Welch was in effect carrying around a hundred pounds of extra weight with him wherever he went, probably wrecking his coronary arteries, all because Timothy McVeigh did something unspeakably evil. Without realizing what he was doing, Bud Welch was "punishing" McVeigh by allowing McVeigh to take over his life.

Then came the day when it dawned on Bud that he was punishing himself far more than he was punishing McVeigh, and that in punishing Timothy McVeigh he was turning himself into exactly what he most despised about McVeigh. Only then did the process of forgiveness and healing begin for him. He stopped asking what sort of person McVeigh was, and started asking, instead, what sort of person Bud Welch wanted to be. In the process, he took back control of his life.

If our inner pharmacy is going to promote healing, it's going to have to make use of the chemical pathways that promote healing in our bodies. As we've learned, one of these routes is the stress/relaxation pathway. When the good chemicals from the inner pharmacy arrive at that pathway, we'd like the road to be clear. We don't want it clogged with heavy traffic carrying extra stress hormones to raise our blood pressures and shut down our immune systems. Faced with that sort of gridlock, how can we expect our inner pharmacy to get its job done?

Any program of self-healing ought to include at some point a forgiveness inventory based on this question: Is there anything in my life that I have resisted forgiving up till now, so that without consciously realizing it, I might be carrying around with me a load of rage that is preventing me from being as healthy as I can be?

Sweating the Small Stuff

The crime from which Bud Welch suffered was truly heinous. Still, many of the actions we refuse to forgive are much less consequential, and indeed can be so minor, it would never occur to us that forgiveness is even an issue. Consider Sid.

Sid's Headache

This story was told by the late Dr. Hiram Curry. For many years, Dr. Curry was head of a nationally recognized family practice training program in Charleston, South Carolina, though his own training was in neurology, not family practice. Toward the end of his career, Dr. Curry wanted to use his training to help patients with common diseases, and so he decided to focus on headache. As he put it, "A medical student can diagnose a brain tumor, and an intern can diagnose a migraine; so I spent all my time on tension headaches." Dr. Curry became the local court of last appeal for headaches that no other doctor could figure out. He attributed his success to the amount of time he was willing to spend talking with each patient to get the full story of the headache.

One of Curry's patients, an accountant whom we'll call "Sid," had been suffering from very severe, incapacitating headaches almost daily for about four years. The usual headache remedies hardly touched them at all, and numerous medical tests had all been negative.

Dr. Curry started to talk with Sid about the headaches and soon discovered that they struck almost every day when he returned home from work. Curry figured that information would be the "smoking gun" he needed. He knew many headache sufferers who endured on-the-job stress; they usually arrived at work pain-free but had developed a raging headache by quitting time. He was also familiar with many people under family stress; they came home without a headache, then had a real humdinger after being at home for an hour or two.

Sid's story simply didn't fit into either of these categories, since cross-examination by Dr. Curry failed to turn up any major stressors either at work or within Sid's family. Still, it seemed on close questioning that he left work fine yet was suffering with an intense headache by the time he got home.

So Dr. Curry next had Sid describe, step-by-step, his afternoon journey from work back home. Sid told Curry that his office was only about six blocks away from his house, and he liked walking to work and back. The headache seemed to hit Sid at the very moment he approached his front gate and entered his yard.

Still puzzled, Dr. Curry was now grasping at anything. "Sid," he said, "at that minute you turn into your front gate from the sidewalk, what do you see in front of you?"

"I see that— *tree*." Sid almost spat out the word as his face reddened with anger.

"It didn't require much genius," Dr. Curry later recalled, "to urge him to tell me more about the tree." The tree, as it turned out, had been planted by Sid's next door neighbor about five years previously. It was a *big* tree. The tree extended two feet over the property line into Sid's yard. He'd measured it himself when the neighbor wasn't around. "That son-of-a-gun," he sputtered on, "to just go and plant that huge tree on my property, without so much as a by-your-leave!" As the story of the tree came out, Sid started to get a headache on the spot. It was obvious he was still seething about this tree every bit as much as the day it was planted.

"So," said Dr. Curry, "what does your neighbor have to say for himself?"

"I don't know. I never talked to him about it."

"Come again?"

"Look, Doctor, I'm the kind of guy who doesn't make waves. I respect my neighbors and expect them to respect me. If it was me, I'd be sure to keep any of my stuff on my property, and no neighbor would ever have to tell me to do that. I figure it should be the same with him. Besides, the sort of guy who would go and smack down this huge tree on my side of the line, what sort of guy is that anyway? Why should I talk to a bozo like that?"

Dr. Curry sent Sid home with one prescription for his headache, and that was to talk to the neighbor about the tree, without fail, and to come back and report in two weeks. The man who appeared for the second visit was a very different Sid.

"Dr. Curry," he beamed, "you won't believe what happened. I talked to my neighbor just like you said. I didn't want to, but I did it anyway. And you know what? He had no idea the tree was over the property line. He thought the line was in a completely different place. And you know what else? He actually offered then and there to go and cut it down! That huge tree! Just like that! Well, how could I make him do that? It's such a big tree and perfectly healthy. You don't just destroy a tree that way. So of course I told him that it was all right and the tree could stay. So he just apologized again and said he wished I had come and talked to him sooner."

"I don't think I need to tell you," Dr. Curry concluded, "that Sid's headaches totally disappeared after that conversation and never returned."

Learning to Forgive Yourself

When we study ourselves to see if there are negative feelings that could obstruct healing, we must be sure to include lack of forgiveness of ourselves, because one very natural human reaction to getting sick is to blame ourselves for it.

As I've said, feeling in control is a critical aspect of a healthy life, and one way to turn on a sluggish inner pharmacy is to take some actions which restore our own sense of mastery over our lives in the face of illness. Unfortunately, one way of feeling in control can be deciding that I must have done this to myself; it wasn't just fate or randomness that made me ill.

In the short run, "I made myself sick" could be construed as a healthy move, since it restores a sense of mastery over my life. But suppose I continue for months, even years, to become really angry at myself for how stupidly I messed up my life by getting sick. I could end up feeling as deep a rage against myself as against any other person I feel may have injured me. In such a case, my accumulated (and usually quite unconscious) rage could form a huge barrier against any healing from my inner pharmacy. I might initially get an ounce or two of extra help from my new sense of control, but, in the long run, that small positive effect is far outweighed by several tons of fury. In these circumstances, learning how to forgive yourself for having gotten sick is just as important a forgiveness task as learning how to forgive someone else.

Suppose that Chuck has to take medication for his diabetes, knows that smoking is an absolute disaster especially for diabetics, and has been told repeatedly that he should exercise. Let's also suppose Chuck constantly forgets to take his medicines, hasn't even tried to quit smoking, and sits on the couch all day. After a number of years go by, we can imagine that Chuck will develop long-term consequences of untreated diabetes, say eye or kidney damage. Imagine Chuck, in his present state of misery, feeling guilty about his past behavior, and blaming himself for what happened.

If Chuck blames himself and feels guilty for what he hasn't done, it would be a reasonable reaction, since there's an obvious, direct link between what he did to himself and his eventual outcome. I am not suggesting, by urging you to avoid judge-and-blame, that I am in favor of totally irresponsible behavior.

But now let's turn this example around. Chuck, having suffered bodily damage from diabetes, has now learned his lesson. What are we to advise him? To keep looking back and blaming himself over and over again? To become enraged at how stupid he had been? Or to move forward and see what he can do, right now, to become and remain somewhat healthier for the rest of his life—at least refusing to pile up even more damage on top of what has occurred? I'd rather Chuck move forward. After all, if he's very angry at himself and feels that he's a low-down, no-good loser, it's highly unlikely that he's going to make much headway toward being healthier. Even in Chuck's much more extreme case, some sort of self-forgiveness may be a major component in his (partial) healing.

Here's an example in which forgiveness of others and forgiveness of self turned out to be closely linked.

Chad's Chronic Pain

Forty-year-old Chad was hit by a car as a teenager and became paralyzed from a broken back as a result. He's been in a wheelchair ever since. For years he worked hard in a high-pressure job. After a serious bout of depression, he realized his family was able to get by on his wife's earnings plus his own disability funds. He quit his job, admitting frankly that perhaps he had been pushing himself harder than he ought. "I was trying to be the 'super-crip'" was how he put it. He thought maybe that was a factor in bringing on his depression.

Two years ago, some pain developed in Chad's arms, which he uses a great deal to compensate for the lack of use of his legs. At first it seemed like nothing more serious than tendinitis, but it persisted and even worsened, despite a variety of medical and surgical treatments and consultations with pain specialists. Whatever the original cause, the arm pain had become a chronic problem with which Chad was going to have to try to live.

Chad's family physician, Dr. Holmes, had always been concerned that there was a psychological component to Chad's pain and worried about a recurrence of the depression, although Chad had shown improvement on a low-dose antidepressant. Nevertheless, the improvement was very limited, and he still had severe problems with his pain. As more time passed, Dr. Holmes recalled the words of a counselor who had seen Chad a few years back: "He seems like one of the angriest people I have ever met."

So Dr. Holmes started to talk to Chad about the anger, and quite a lot of feelings began to emerge. For the first time, Chad was able to verbalize to Dr. Holmes how enraged he still was at the driver who had hit him and caused his paralysis. In addition, the man had managed to evade legal responsibility and Chad's father, who had not been well off financially, had ended up with costs for Chad's rehabilitation he simply couldn't handle. "I can never forgive that bastard," Chad fumed. "If there is anything that's totally despicable, it's running away from your responsibilities. I try to be sure that I always meet my responsibilities and I want to raise my kids to be that way, too. How can I forgive that guy? It would be the same as telling my kids that whether you meet your responsibilities or run away doesn't matter."

Dr. Holmes persisted in his counseling role during several months, being sure to give Chad breathing spells in between their visits so as not to push him further than he was ready to go at any time. Gently he tried to probe the obvious association between the anger and the pain. Could it be that part of the reason for Chad's inability to release his anger at the driver was his never forgiving himself for not being employed and depending upon his wife's income? Was he actually projecting the charge of "irresponsibility" onto the driver so that he would not have to face his own anger or loathing at his own behavior?

Chad's language, when Dr. Holmes was first able to get him to see the germ of this idea, was not fit for reprinting. But after fuming for a few weeks, he was actually able to cry at a later visit and to start to admit the difficulty of no longer being his family's breadwinner, and how he still secretly reproached himself, years later, for "just sitting at home while my wife earns the paycheck."

Only after Chad was able to admit his own feelings about himself was he able to tackle the problem of forgiving the driver and letting go of all the rage he had accumulated. When he eventually reached the point of completion, he expressed to Dr. Holmes his amazement at how much "lighter" he suddenly felt. After a few more months Chad and Dr. Holmes were astonished at how little pain medication he needed to manage his symptoms.

Forgiveness can be an extremely powerful healing tool to assist the inner pharmacy—but only when it's real.

The Difficult Work of True Forgiveness

Today, forgiveness is a popular concept in mind-body and self-help circles. Ann Landers even writes an annual forgiveness column. I feel the very popularity of forgiveness explains some of the situations where it seems not to work. It's easy to forgive other people verbally, when our deep-down feelings and attitudes have not changed. As opposed to Chad's case, Sid's grievance against his neighbor and his tree was rather superficial, once he became aware of it. As soon as he confronted the real situation, his forgiveness was as immediate as it was genuine. He didn't have to spend years in counseling to figure out how to forgive.

Suppose, in contrast, that Sid's neighbor had done something as bad to him as the driver of the car did to Chad—and did it consciously from highly suspect motives. Sid might, after reading an Ann Landers column, decide it would be a good idea to forgive the man and might even say the words out loud and feel temporarily better. But would he really have forgiven him? It might be only months later, when we found his headaches hadn't diminished, that we'd realize he'd gone through the motions but hadn't gotten down deep to where his true feelings lay.

I have known patients who thought they'd completely forgiven others (or themselves) five or six times; only to undergo a profound and thorough change in their feelings and attitudes the final time. In cases where the lack of forgiveness is buried so deeply, counseling is often necessary to get to the root of the problem.

Desire, Forgiveness, and Meaning

We have seen how ambivalent feelings about getting better, as well as lack of forgiveness, can be barriers to the effective working of the inner pharmacy. In keeping with our model, we should make note of what each of these factors has to do with meaning. Clearly, if we rid ourselves of the ambivalent feelings standing in the way of our desire to be healthy, we change the meaning of the treatment for our illness. The treatment was previously a threat, because it might possibly rob us of the attention we craved from others, or it might make us face up to even more serious changes we needed to make but had been avoiding. Now it has only positive meaning for us because we truly want to get better.

Forgiveness has less to do with the meaning of the specific illness or treatment and much more to do with the meaning of our lives. Forgiveness has to do with what type of person we want to be. It also involves who has control over our lives: Paradoxically, the more we refuse to forgive others, the more we hand over control of our lives and its meaning.

Next, we need to look at how we can work with stories to help our inner pharmacy to do more for our health.

THIRTEEN

Enhancing Meaning Through Stories

"'I would ask you to remember only this one thing,' said Badger. 'The stories people tell have a way of taking care of them. If stories come to you, care for them. And learn to give them away where they are needed. Sometimes a person needs a story more than food to stay alive.'"

—Barry Lopez, 1993

The next step in harnessing the placebo response and the inner pharmacy for your own health is to remain constantly aware that these processes depend heavily on the meaning you attach to the illness and the treatment. By now, you know that positive meaning has several components: an explanation that makes sense; care or concern shown by others; and a sense of greater control or mastery over the illness and its symptoms. I've also described *telling stories* as the most basic human method of assigning meaning to puzzling or threatening events.

The Work of Story Work

Tim's Rash/Tim's Boss

Dr. Bill Hankins, who trained in the same family residency practice program as I did, liked to tell this story. It concerned a thirty-four-year-old patient named "Tim" who came to see Bill several times during a couple of months because of a bothersome skin rash. Initially, Tim's condition was frustrating since Hankins couldn't recognize the rash as representing any specific disease, and the general skin remedies he prescribed didn't alleviate the constant itch Tim reported. On the third or fourth visit, Bill determined to try a new tack and act on his belief in the mind-body connection by asking Tim to describe in general what had been going on in his life during the last several months.

Tim talked a little about his family and home, but, when he switched the subject to work, it became evident that he and his boss were having a serious conflict which seemed to have worsened around the time the rash appeared. After listening to Tim rant on about his superior's maddening mannerisms and boundless shortcomings, Dr. Hankins had an inspiration; the next time Tim stopped to get his breath, Bill observed, "It sounds like he really gets under your skin."

As Dr. Hankins tells the story, "If Tim had been a character in a cartoon, you would have seen a little lightbulb start to glow over his head as he made the connection. He immediately agreed that the timing was perfect to explain the symptom. The rash disappeared shortly after and never bothered him again."

This anecdote is definitely an example of story work. When Tim left Dr. Hankins's office that day, he had a radically different narrative of his rash. The revised story imbued his symptoms with a much different meaning, and that new meaning, in itself, produced an almost magical cure. Yet Tim's case is an extremely limited example of what we want to accomplish in this chapter, since the new story was almost exclusively Dr. Hankins's creation. Granted, Tim instantly recognized its pertinence, but he played almost no role in devising it.

By contrast, the story work we will be discussing here makes you the author of your own life story, including your health and illness. That's as it should be; who could be more qualified to write your biography than you? I've tried on a number of occasions to hand patients ready-made stories and must admit I've very seldom had Bill Hankins's success. In my experience, the stories that work best in terms of healing are ones in which the patient has been intimately involved as author or coauthor.

The successful story work you can do on your own, or with the right help, requires finding a way to translate the three components of the meaning model into your story work. This involves three steps:

1. Tell yourself the full story of your illness and locate this story within your life's story (your biography).
2. See who will listen to your story.
3. Think about ways to rewrite the story so that it has a better ending.

Now, let's look at each one in turn, beginning with creating the story itself.

Story Making

Tell yourself the full story of your illness and locate this story within your life's story (your biography).

The first step in helping yourself deal with an illness is to form the best explanation you can. This demands telling its story: how it first came into your life; what seemed to cause it; whether it is like or unlike other things that happened to you in the past; and the changes you sustained as you proceeded to deal with it.

Here's an illustrative anecdote:

What Does It Mean to Break Your Hip?

Dr. Jeffrey Borkan and colleagues at the University of Massachusetts were interested in the thoughts of elderly people who suffer from broken hips. They interviewed patients who'd had steel pins surgically inserted in their hips, and who were now recovering in a rehabilitation center. Borkan and colleagues also followed the healing process of these patients for six months after the operations.

The study was conducted in the manner of anthropologists observing a person's culture, with very detailed, personalized interviews. All the patients were asked to tell the story of how their hips came to be broken and what had happened as a result. The purpose of the interviews was to get to the root of the question, "What does all this *mean* to you?"

When the researchers looked at all the collected stories, they found they fell essentially into two categories. One group of patients told fairly simple, matter-of-fact stories that basically went: "I was healthy and going about my usual business, but then I had an accident, fell, and broke my hip."

The other group presented more convoluted, fatalistic narratives: "First I came down with such-and-such a disease, and then as my health got worse, I got these other problems, and then more things happened to me, and finally I was so sick that I couldn't manage to walk without getting dizzy or weak, and so finally I fell and broke my hip."

At the start of the research, there didn't seem to be any obvious medical difference between the two groups of patients. By its conclusion, Dr. Borkan and his colleagues were fascinated to see that the first group—the "healthy, had an accident" group—healed up after surgery substantially faster than the "already damaged" group.

We would obviously have to do more research to see whether working with the negative patients to help them revise their stories would have an effect on their physical outcome.

In any case, it's important to remember that there's no simple formula for how to tell the story of your illness because for this to be a healing experience, the story must be truly *yours*.

How Do I Decide What Story Is Right for Me?

Just because it's your job to create your own story won't stop other people from trying, with the best of intentions, to tell you *their* story of your illness, insisting it's the correct version. Your physician, of course, will tell you the medical story: the diagnosis, prescribed treatment, and her best available estimation of the future outcome of your condition. Then your neighbor or cousin will tell you that the doctor doesn't know what she's talking about, and that your symptoms are just like her friend Sara's when she had gallstones; so of course your problem is gallstones, and you need surgery. If you talk to other people with your same problem—especially if they have formed a special organization for patients with that disease—they may tell you how they coped with it and how in their view the ideal patient in their organization behaves.

You are free to make use of any or all of this information in telling your own story of your illness, but you are not bound by it. The story must be what you think happened and what makes the most sense to you. It wouldn't be surprising, especially if the illness has been a major disruption in your life, if it takes you weeks, months, or even years to be able to give a full account.

As hard as it might be to construct the story of your illness, the work is not yet done. If this is truly to be your story of your own illness, it's a chapter or a series of chapters in the entire story which is your life. We won't know what this illness means to you until we can see it placed correctly in the context of your biography. Some illness accounts are temporary interruptions in your life story. After they subside, you go back about your business. Other stories, especially of major illnesses like diabetes or major disabilities like a stroke, alter the whole flow and direction of your autobiography: You become a different person, leading a different life. Especially in this latter case, it is critical to view the story nested inside your autobiography to see precisely what the illness means to you.

Arthur Frank, a sociologist who survived cancer and a heart attack while still in his thirties, has spent a lot of time studying the more complex illness stories of those whose lives will never be the same again. He is sensitive to the need not to create strict categories and to be careful to listen to each individual's story on its own merits and discern its own structure. With that caution, he says that he can describe generally three types of stories that are commonly told about serious chronic illness.

Chaos, Restitution, and the Quest

The chaos story is a strange mix of story and nonstory. It is what we relate when, overwhelmed by the illness, we can't find the right words to express our terror. For the afflicted person, it reflects not only fear, but also the confusion and general tangle of emotions he is bound up in. Right now he can't see beyond that tangle. Such a narrative is difficult for others to listen to and tends to drive them away to less threatening ground. Fortunately for most ill people who survive for any period of time without major brain damage, this stage of storytelling is temporary.

The *restitution story* is the type of narrative doctors prefer to relate, and that most of us, at least in the early stages of serious life-threatening illness, prefer to hear: after the proper treatment, everything will be fixed, and the illness will be just an unpleasant memory. Doctors like to tell a version of the restitution story in which they get to be the heroes: The patient submits to standard medical therapy; the therapy works; and everyone lives happily ever after.

On the other hand, critics of modern medicine tend to tell a different version of the restitution story in which the conventional physicians try their standard, ultimately ineffective treatments; the patient grows worse and more desperate, finally deciding to take matters into his own hands. Eventually, he finds his way to an alternative healer who has the right nutritional formula or herbal remedy; the patient is finally cured; the doctors are amazed and chagrined; and everyone lives happily ever after. Still, the bottom line in both cases is "not to worry" because the patient will eventually be able to get on with his life, without the illness leaving a permanent mark on his identity.

Restitution stories make for great storytelling, but there's a problem with them. Because we are all going to die someday, restitution stories must some of the time be false.

The good news is that modern medicine has made chronic disease survivable when it cannot be cured. A hundred years ago, many youthful people died from infections which today would be prevented or reversed. Those who came down with diseases like coronary disease, cancer, or diabetes usually succumbed in the illness's early stages. Today, we still cannot cure those diseases, but it's now possible to extend life until the very late stages of the illness. The bad news is that science has not been able to make our lives the same as they would have been without the disease. We still have things that we have to do (taking insulin shots daily), and things we can't do that we'd like to (climbing stairs without getting short of breath), which remind us every day that we're living with a disease. This means that something different from a restitution story is what will ultimately make the most sense for us.

Quest stories are Frank's last and most interesting category of narratives about chronic serious illness. The quest story is similar to the long fairy tales that were read to us as children, in which the hero sets out to accomplish a task like slaying a dragon or rescuing a maiden in distress. He may or may not be able to accomplish this task, but he sustains a series of adventures along the way. The adventures may distract the hero from his task for a time. The adventures may better prepare him for the task: Helpful folks befriend him and give him various magic spells and other tools which he'll need when facing the dragon. The adventures may even be critical to completing the task because the hero proves himself worthy of the final challenge by first overcoming more modest ones.

Still, the main message of the quest story is that by the end, the hero has changed. He is no longer the brash, callow youth who began the quest; he has been toughened and deepened by his experiences. If he accomplishes the task, it is due to the new skills and wisdom he brings to it. If he does not, it is because he sees the task from a new vantage point, realizing that his youthful ambition was actually a foolish fancy, and that what will genuinely bring fulfillment to his life is something quite different from what he first imagined. Remember Dorothy in *The Wizard of Oz* deciding in the end, "There's no place like home."

The concept of the quest story may sound overly romanticized. But if you accept Arthur Frank's interpretation, you'll realize it's critical in relieving suffering. Frank's version goes something like this: "My life is a journey. I am headed some place, for some purpose. There are things I want to do and accomplish. Along the way, I have been struck by this chronic illness. I have been slowed down and diverted from my quest by this illness, and now is the time for me to get going again. My current job is to find a way to put this illness in perspective. It happened to me, and it is part of my life from now on, but it is not my whole life and it should not, in the end, keep me from my quest."

For a person who may never fully recover from a serious chronic illness, a quest story is often the most meaningful and satisfying story to tell. In Frank's view, many people with such chronic illnesses suffer terribly, in part because they are still trying to cling to restitution stories which are obviously not working, and have not yet figured out how to tell a quest story. If there is anything our society should be doing for people with serious chronic illnesses today, it would be to help them figure out better stories to tell when their existing stories seem not to be working.

Try to recall how many TV and newspaper stories you've seen recently announcing a new miracle "breakthrough" in the cure of some disease—always with the fine print adding that it may be years before this wonderful new treatment will actually be available for human use. If the popular media focused less on restitution stories and showed us more examples of helpful quest stories and adaptations, think how much more the quality of life of people with chronic illness would be improved.

Dr. Frank offers his categories without judging which type of story is appropriate for any particular person with an illness. Different stories may work at different stages. To take an example we've used before: A person who develops cancer, overwhelmed with the news about the diagnosis, might first tell a chaos story; then tell a restitution story when she starts treatment for as long as the treatment is working; then tell a new chaos story when she discovers that the cancer is spreading despite the treatment; and finally tell a quest story when she comes to terms with the fact that she will eventually die of her cancer, but that in the meantime she intends to live as fully and as meaningfully as she can, seeking medical or complementary treatment that will help her to function day-to-day rather than continuing vainly to seek a cure. For this individual, the restitution story was "wrong" in the end; but similarly the quest story would have been premature when there was a reasonable hope that the curative treatment would work.

Storytelling and Listening

See who will listen to your story.

Arthur Frank attributes the suffering of the incurably ill only in part to the difficulty in telling a quest story, or whatever other story would be most meaningful for the individual. Another source of suffering, as we've noted, is the isolation the sick experience when others are too threatened to listen. Our analysis of the placebo response shows that people do much better when they feel care and concern from those around them, in part by knowing they are being listened to and that their meaningful story of illness is thus being validated. The need to make sense of what is happening to us when we are sick is a very basic one. Having no one to listen to us as we try to tell the story leads to a deep sense of loneliness and despair. To be unlistened to is like being evicted from the human community.

I can't stress this point about validation strongly enough. I'm sure all physicians have seen a case like this: A patient has puzzling symptoms, maybe so strange that they seem to be psychosomatic. After many months or even years of testing and study, the physicians finally make a diagnosis of an obscure cancer. One would think that the patient would be devastated by this "bad news." Yet the patient is strangely relieved and calm. He says, "See! All along I told you that something was wrong, and now we have proof that I was right." The great relief of suffering that comes with validation of what he had been going through all this time outweighs for him the negative impact of the dreadful diagnosis.

Arthur Frank goes so far as to argue that the giving and listening to the testimony of the ill is an important social practice by which, in the end, all of us are healed. The sick are healed because being listened to affirms their essential humanity. The rest of us will someday be healed by those stories—little as we realize it today—because someday we will be sick too, and will need reassurance that other humans have coped with that sort of sickness and survived to tell about it.

But how can you ensure that others will listen to you? After all, some sick people are also friendless and far from their families. It's also the case that many ill persons' behavior makes it harder for even those who love them to listen to their stories. To be sick is often to be self-absorbed, to live in a shrunken world, to think that your symptoms and complaints are all-encompassing. Telling the story of your sickness in a way that brings meaning to the experience and locates the illness within your autobiography is quite different from merely complaining on and on about your stomachache or your constipation or your itching. When we are sick, we must ask ourselves if we're behaving as the type of person whose story others will find worthwhile and want to listen to.

Mitch Albom's book, *Tuesdays with Morrie*, has become a longtime bestseller despite its apparently depressing theme—a former student, now a journalist, making weekly trips to listen to his old college professor stricken with Lou Gehrig's disease talk about what it means to be dying. I hope one of the reasons for the deserved popularity of the book is the model that the professor offers of how to tell the *true* story of his illness, resisting any temptation to prettify something if it's really unpleasant while making the story and its teller interesting and valuable.

Searching Honesty

We can all ponder how to create interesting stories and how to make our listeners feel more valued because they're hearing us. The difference between a story worth listening to and mere self-absorbed complaining lies primarily in searching honesty. The person who is merely griping is basically manipulative: He wants you to feel sorry for him and to pay attention to him, but doesn't want to admit it; nor does he seek to explore why he feels the need for pity. By contrast, somebody like Morrie is genuinely frank, attempting to put his illness in the context of the meaning of his life, revealing his deep respect for the listener by honestly and thoroughly explaining himself. The listener is bound to feel valued and eager to come back again.

What if you've tried your best, yet you still find yourself all alone with no one to listen to your story? One thing you can do is find others who need to be listened to. You have experienced, at first hand, how miserable a person can be when she is ill and no one is around to listen.

Might that not make you especially suitable to ensure that others don't have to suffer the way you have? Doing good for others—even if no one listens to your own story—will at least have the beneficial (and healing) result of getting you socially reconnected. If you take the plunge and genuinely go out looking for others to help, I very much doubt that you yourself will remain long without listeners.

Story Revising

Think about ways to rewrite the story so that it has a better ending.

Our lives are unfolding stories. Some of the story is written for us by forces outside our control. We didn't get to choose our parents or the hometown in which we grew up. But we have at least some power to write the story the way we want it to come out. This is especially true when it comes to the attitudes we take toward events or the meaning we attribute to those events. Let's see how this worked for Hank.

Hank's Migraines

"Hank," forty-one, became my patient when one of my partners left the practice. During the more than ten years that he'd been seeing my partner, Hank had suffered from severe migraine headaches that came on at least once a week and sometimes lasted for three days. He'd tried all the usual treatments and preventives for migraine (the list filled an entire page) and consulted with several major headache clinics. Each proposed remedy either didn't work or caused dangerous side effects, with a single exception: narcotic pain relievers taken once the headache had begun. Over the years, Hank had learned to inject himself with the powerful narcotic Demerol and each month received a prescription for twelve injections. He sometimes could get the edge off the headache if he took Vicodin, a less powerful narcotic which came in pill form, so he used about 120 of those every month as well. My partner had kept him on this schedule, which he followed religiously. My choice seemed to be between continuing to prescribe the medications or having Hank constantly running to a hospital emergency room with a killer migraine. It was not a great case for a new doctor to take over. But I felt it would be inhumane to take away his medications and just let him suffer.

Finally, I decided to tell him that, at least for a while, I'd continue the prescriptions if he'd allow us to monitor his drug use carefully on a monthly basis. Meanwhile, I tried to get to know my patient better. Married with two teenaged children, Hank was presently working toward a Ph.D. at the university where I practice. During our monthly visits, I encouraged him to tell me the story of his headaches, and gradually a picture emerged.

Hank revealed two things about his headaches which seemed to provide me with some clues for action. First, the headaches had a very clear meaning for him: "unemployable." He had been fired from an earlier job due to his headaches, which had caused him to take an unreasonable number of sick days. He was diligently pursuing his degree, but saw himself doing graduate work because it was interesting and fulfilling, and because he had started it and meant to finish it, not because he had great hopes for a career later on. It also turned out that his in-laws were on his case about this, basically telling his wife that she'd married a real loser, and ridiculing his wasting money on graduate school.

The other thing Hank told me was that the onset of a migraine panicked him. He knew he could take his Demerol shots and relieve some of the pain, but he also appreciated the fact that, as soon as he took the shot, he was essentially out of commission for the rest of the day. He had come to the office several times with what appeared to us to be very severe headaches, and I had offered him a shot of Demerol. He always refused, because he'd driven to the office and didn't want to risk driving home on Demerol; he preferred to tough it out until he got home. What panicked him most was the possibility of a migraine's starting up when he absolutely had to do something that could not be postponed and which required narcotic-free alertness.

When I asked Hank for more detail, it turned out that his most intense panic occurred at the first signs of the headache. In fact, he'd frequently managed to complete a task, headache and all. From these observations, I concluded he had not one, but two problems: the headache, and his terror of the headache.

As we talked this over, it became clear that Hank certainly didn't like taking the narcotics and dreamed of someday being free of them, so he was willing to try anything I might have in mind.

First we worked on the panic reaction, with my reminding him how often he'd fought through the headache when he had no other choice. Yet he'd never really given himself credit for this accomplishment because his self-testimony was still a story of failure. I encouraged him to concentrate on those successful episodes and try to figure out what had been unique about them.

Next, I suggested, "Try thinking of a message you can tell yourself, over and over again, when you begin to get one of the really bad migraines. A message that will remind you of your past successes and reduce your panic. Something that will say to you, 'I know I'm going to have a migraine and that it'll hurt a lot, but there is no reason I need to have all this panic in addition.'" I felt a saying he invented himself was much more likely to work than one I handed to him. Initially, he wasn't sure what the right verbal formula was, though he was excited about the idea. I made coming up with a saying his homework assignment for the next month. When he did, I advised him to practice it for a month and see what happened.

There was nothing magical about the "mantra" Hank finally arrived at. He simply repeated over and over that he knew the headaches weren't going to kill him and that he could accomplish important tasks first and take his medicine later. He seemed to believe it in a way he hadn't before. As proof, he reported when a few months had passed that—although the headaches were still there—he'd reduced his panic reaction by about 75 percent.

I'd love to take credit for what happened next, but the main forces at work were totally outside of my control. While Hank was finishing his Ph.D., the graduate department was starting up a new project which entailed sending faculty on the road to teach classes at distant sites around the state. Even though the faculty knew about Hank's migraines, they offered him the job of directing the new project—a doubly scary prospect, since he had to work forty hours a week (at least), drive long distances, and be ready to work at the top of his form once he reached his destination. If he arrived in a city three hours away and started to get a migraine, he would still have to teach his two-hour class before he could give himself a shot of Demerol.

Hank took the job, determined not to miss work due to migraines; by now he was much more confident that he could handle the headaches with little or no panic. He was starting to rewrite the story of his life with migraines in a more positive way. I meanwhile continued renewing the narcotic prescriptions each month, actually fighting off Hank's requests that we start to cut down. We'd have plenty of time, I told him, to reduce his dosages once he got into the swing of his new job and adjusted to his travel schedule. What I wanted to avoid was his taking too much responsibility all at once, possibly failing, and then going into a discouraging tailspin.

After a year on his new job, Hank was very proud to report he'd missed only one day of work due to headaches. He had many success stories to tell from the year of his victory over his headaches—and his bosses were so obviously pleased with his performance, they were eager to give him more responsibility.

At this writing, Hank is on his way to Germany to start a new international phase of his project. We've agreed that once he gets back from that trip, we're going to start gradually reducing the Demerol and Vicodin. So far, Hank's headaches have not gotten noticeably better, but I am fully confident that with time they will indeed reduce in intensity and frequency. More importantly, even if they don't, Hank knows that he can live with them in a way he couldn't before.

How can one go about rewriting one's own story as Hank did so that it has a better, more positive conclusion?

Happy Endings

If I'm sick and read books or stories about other sick people and the stories they have told about their own illnesses, I will definitely learn certain lessons. What I will not come away with is a ready-made set of meanings I can simply paste onto my own illness to become instantly happier and to get an instant surge in my inner pharmacy.

There are a few people who allow the rest of the world to tell them what their lives mean. Most of us, however, are willing to struggle to find the meaning of our own lives, even if the rest of the world is trying to hand us a very lovely story. In other words, if I'm in despair over my future because of my illness, reading a lot of uplifting stories will not, by itself, turn me into an optimist, nor will it suddenly alleviate all my symptoms due to an upsurge in the placebo response.

If I am genuinely searching for meaning in my life, and I am genuinely open to the idea that things could get better only if I work at it and allow it to happen, then listening to these other stories may trigger an act of imagination, in which I could start to see a range of different future possibilities for myself. Instead of devising a single ending to the story—probably a very discouraging one—I might start to ask myself if I need to look around more, look inside myself more, and see if there are not some strengths and some resources left that could make a real difference in how my story comes out.

To explore further the importance of revising our stories, I'm going to turn to some examples of people facing death. I think it's vitally important—and in fact extremely healthy—to look not only at optimistic, uplifting narratives but at this type of story as well.

Storytelling at the End of Life

As I've said, story work means placing our testimony about the illness or health problem within the larger context of the story of our lives, in such a way that both the illness story and the larger life story acquire greatest meaning. An autobiography is ultimately the narrative of a *complete* life, and we must face the fact that our life stories are not complete until we come to the ending. There are valuable lessons we can learn about how to construct a meaningful and healing story by looking at a person who is actually facing death.

Finally, I want to anticipate a bit of the "mystery" of the placebo response: When we can best accept the fact that some day we are going to die, we have freed up our inner pharmacies to do their best and most complete work.

I'll try to explain more fully what I mean by this in the last chapter. For now, let's just think of how our acceptance of death relates to the stress pathway. Our modern culture, by its pervasive message that dying is the very worst thing that can happen to us, stresses us with unrelieved fear of death. When we reduce that level of stress by accepting death as a natural part of a meaningful and satisfying life, we free the biochemical pathways to let the inner pharmacy operate unimpeded.

In this chapter, I could have ignored all talk of death and dying and presented you exclusively with "happy endings." But if I confined myself only to superficially "uplifting" stories, I would actually be undermining your full potential for health.

With all these reasons in mind, let's turn to an example. Suppose I happen to be dying of advanced cancer. Perhaps my story of suffering has me dying alone in great pain, and my death dominates my thoughts so much that day-to-day activities seem hardly worth doing. Instead I could start thinking about what I hope to accomplish with whatever days I have left. I could make a list of my unfinished business. Some of it—like taking up Rollerblading, for instance—I can quickly cross off. Other things such as making amends with people I have estranged or offended or making some tapes of recollections of my early life to leave for my children and grandchildren might be possible to achieve.

As I begin to think about getting something accomplished in my remaining time on earth, the days start to take on a new meaning. There begins to be a sense of hope about my life. This will be enhanced further as I learn more about pain control and find out that I need not fear being in severe pain at the end of life. This hope is not hope for a miracle cure or a long survival; it is a quite realistic hope that I can do certain concrete things and give added meaning to my last days. It is the hope that when I am about to die, I will be able to look back with some pride on how I chose to spend my time during these weeks or months.

It will interest you to know that people who work in hospice programs and who regularly deal with patients facing these choices notice that certain things happen. Patients who develop this sort of attitude, and this sort of positive, even if modest, hope, often "die well." They seem to get the most satisfaction out of their days, handle their pain and other unpleasant symptoms better than other patients, and appear to draw from others the most loving and compassionate support. Although it's hard to predict or to quantify these things, a number of these folks seem to live somewhat longer than predicted. Maybe the enhanced meaning of their lives, the better ending they are writing for their own stories, has an impact on their bodies' inner pharmacies.

The Importance of Story Work: A Summing Up

Story work goes on in families, around the dinner table and elsewhere, just as it always has done since the dawn of humanity. Storytelling as a healing tool, though, is still a rather new idea. Someday people with chronic or terminal illnesses may be able to sign up for story workshops, where trained staff will work with groups of patients, using years of training and experience to help midwife the birth of the right story for each person. Indeed, the best contemporary self-help illness groups of cancer patients and others seem to function that way, without anyone actually calling the process "story work." You might be able to find expert help with this task of working on meaning; or you might find yourself depending on your own resources and those of your circle of family and friends.

Meaning in life is a basic human need, and story work (however sporadic or informal) is the main tool we have for creating personal meaning. Even if I have another forty or fifty years left to live, I will be happier, and I suspect healthier, if I put some of my energy right now into making better sense of what is happening to me by using these tools. Many more people would "die well" today if they had laid the ground for their story work much earlier in life and did not have quite so much catching up to do when death was right around the corner.

Social connection and social isolation are major determinants of how you respond to illness and of whether or not your inner pharmacy comes to your aid. The next chapter will go deeper into the importance of social connections.

FOURTEEN

Maintaining Social Connections

"The tendency when we're ill is to close ourselves off, not let people know. But I don't think we can go off in caves and heal by ourselves. In some mysterious way, it's a communal experience. I think healing is contagious, just like infection."

—Marc Ian Barasch

Two different drugs are used as clot dissolvers in patients having heart attacks. One, which happens to be the more expensive, has in recent years been widely preferred over the less costly medication. Asked why they insist upon the more costly drug, physicians commonly explain that it's slightly more effective. But just how much more? In a major scientific study widely quoted in defense of the expensive drug, the risk of dying was shown to be 7 percent with the cheaper drug and 6 percent with the more expensive one.

In modern medical practice, it's not unusual for a particular drug or surgery to be preferred over another because of such statistics: a difference of merely a few percentage points. So what—in terms of percentage points—are we to make of the comparable importance of social isolation and connectedness in illness and health?

A number of major studies have been done to measure the risk of getting sick or dying if you are socially isolated, and the effect is *not* a few percentage points. In fact, these studies show that social isolation is associated with a two- to three-fold difference in the risk of death or serious illness, especially in older people. That's two hundred or three hundred percentage points difference. Isn't it astounding that American medicine has not made more of this risk factor? In another sense, it's not astounding at all; it's just further evidence of how American medicine tries resolutely to focus on the body and ignore the mind.

Other People as Healing Agents

I can't stress firmly enough what a major difference maintaining social connections can make in the course of an illness. Here's an anecdote to underscore my point:

A Family Gathering

"Daisy," a portly, pleasant-faced woman of seventy-seven, suffered from emphysema as the result of many years of cigarette smoking. She also had what physicians, in days gone by, called "hypochondriasis"—so she'd frequently come to see me with a wide variety of minor complaints. As a rule, it took only a brief discussion of Daisy's new symptom before she turned the conversation to the subject of her family. It was quite large, but relations between members seemed always to be strained. During each visit, I'd hear that a nephew or grandson was sick or in jail or having serious financial problems; or that a relative was angry at Daisy and not speaking to her for some arcane reason. She seemed to take each incident as a personal criticism. Why, she wondered, couldn't her family be united, content, and pleasant to one another, like the families portrayed in the popular TV shows of the time?

Daisy eventually developed lung cancer. As no treatment was likely to prolong her life, she chose the local home hospice care program as her best option for aid. A nurse came regularly to Daisy's apartment, and we easily controlled the small amount of pain she was having with the appropriate medicines.

I hadn't seen Daisy for a while when I received a call from the hospice nurse who told me Daisy was confined to bed and that Daisy and everyone who had seen her in the last few days was sure she was dying. As often happens when a patient is near death, she was having more trouble with pain, and I felt she probably needed her medication adjusted. I decided to make a home visit the first chance I got, which turned out to be that evening.

To my surprise, when I arrived at the apartment, I found it difficult to make my way through a large crowd of people to get to the bedroom. It seemed that every member of her family—at least the ones not currently in jail—had come to visit once they'd received word she was dying. I found Daisy looking weak, but absolutely beaming because of all the love and attention she was receiving.

Since the nurse and I had discussed how to adjust the medication to make Daisy's last hours as comfortable as possible, I checked in the next morning to see how things were going. Imagine my amazement when the nurse told me Daisy had rallied substantially. The nurse was very experienced and could usually tell with certainty when a patient was near death. This sudden reversal had totally stunned her. Daisy was soon up and about the apartment. On a later home visit, I half-jokingly accused her of enjoying her deathbed family gathering so much that it seemed a real waste to die just then. She just smiled back.

Daisy did succumb a number of weeks later, having, in the interim, received more attention from her family. She managed to prolong her life and improve its quality as well.

I've mentioned that many studies dramatically show the dire effects of social isolation on health. Now it's time to ask the big question: Will your risk of dying or getting worse go down—and your inner pharmacy fire up—if you become more socially connected?

The few studies that have been done tend to be rather promising. The good news for animal lovers is that caring for a pet can reduce the health risk of social isolation.

We have talked about one of the most important steps in making meaning out of your experience of illness: finding someone to listen to your story. It makes sense that the more socially connected you are, the easier it will be to get listened to when you most need it. So avoiding social isolation may be very important in maintaining health because it helps in the process of returning meaning to your life; or maybe it's health-giving in some other way. Until we do a lot more research to see which biochemical pathways are activated by social connections, we won't know for sure.

In talking about what to do to maintain and nurture your social connections, both for better health and for general happiness, I must address two groups separately. The first group has no particular reason for being socially isolated, except that other things in life just seemed to take higher priority. The second group has been lonely *and* depressed; their depression is the major cause of their social isolation. Obviously these two groups will need different strategies in order to become connected.

"I've Just Been Too Busy"

A bit of advance planning helps greatly in maintaining strong social connections. Suppose you've been socially isolated for years and then come down with a serious illness. Then you read this book and decide that to enhance the placebo response, you should try to give new, positive meaning to what has happened to you; then what? Maybe you find a social network to join; self-help and support groups that are often created by various disease-focused organizations and medical centers may be effective ways to do this. In fact, if you look around you, you'll have a wide choice of networks from which to choose: your religious community, if you're an active participant; your doctors and nurses; the various formal organizations I've mentioned above; and, of course, your friends and family.

In fact, reviving past social connections is an especially beneficial thing to do for yourself if you want to stay healthy, although this may be a new idea to you. Before now, if asked about things you *ought* to do to stay as healthy as possible, you'd very likely mention eating the right foods and getting exercise. Yet you might never have thought that calling a cousin you hadn't seen for two years but with whom you'd been meaning to get in touch could benefit your health.

I don't mean to suggest that staying healthy is the only reason why you'd want to get socially connected. I trust that there are many other benefits that have nothing to do with health. By nature, people are social animals whose sense of well-being is greatly enhanced by feeling that we belong in a secure place within a familiar social group, especially in today's world, where it's increasingly difficult to maintain this sense of belonging. Many other aspects of our lives compete for our minute-by-minute attention. Friends and loved ones move away. Some people simply have an easier time than others making social connectedness a priority.

If you want to enhance the health-giving effects of maintaining strong social connections, here's what you should be doing all along—well before you get sick—to keep your inner pharmacy working well.

1. Many people think that social connections ought to be spontaneous and become artificial or phony if you have to work at making them happen. This makes no more sense than insisting that exercise ought to be spontaneous—that having to rearrange your schedule to find time to work out somehow makes the exercise bad for you.

   I'll grant you that a focus on relationships takes work and planning. Regardless, most of us could benefit from thinking harder about those social relationships, noting which ones we've been attending to and which we've been neglecting. If we realize, as often happens, that some of the relationships we've let slide are actually quite important to us, we'll make the time to devote to them.
2. As we've discussed, sick people with stories to tell about their reactions to illnesses have something valuable to share and to add to the life of the community. Yet we're more likely, at first, to suspect they'll drain the emotional energy of people who aren't ill. Let's be honest—how many of us, given the choice between going to a party and visiting a sick friend in the hospital, would choose the hospital? That reaction is short-sighted. In the end, visiting the sick friend might actually recharge my emotional batteries much

more than any party—as Mitch Albom found out with Morrie.

3. Real social connections are two-way streets. If you are going to be there for me when I really need you, then I am going to have to be there for you. Some people who find themselves lonely and isolated when they are seriously ill were too busy before ever to be there for others in need.

   If you are socially isolated and want to get reconnected, seek situations in which others need you. Almost always, when you decide to try to give something to others by your human contact and care, you discover quite unexpectedly that you will be getting back even more than what you have given out. Doctors and nurses may not admit it, but that may be why they went into careers in health care, and also why they keep doing it year after year. And no one has to be a trained professional in order to find ways to help. It's very rare for those who have spent years trying to help others to suddenly find themselves socially isolated when they themselves are sick and needy.

4. Some people suffer terribly during serious or terminal illness because of their separation from relatives or friends with whom they were once close. Of course, as we've noted, it's not uncommon for sick people to be shunned by family and friends through no fault of their own. In fact, some of the cases in which this suffering is most severe involve long-time feuds or estrangements which have gradually become set in concrete, since no one made the right moves to mend fences while time was passing. It's also not unusual for the sick person to say, "I'm the one who's dying, so it's up to him to apologize, if he really cares—otherwise I don't want to hear from him." These cases remind us that one special form of social isolation which seems to cause great suffering for the sick and dying is related to lack of forgiveness.

Social Isolation and Depression

An inability to make connections may also be due to the fact that a person may for years have been suffering from depression. Depression and social isolation tend to go together for a couple of reasons. Depressed people lack the energy to maintain social contacts. Because it can be depressing to be around a depressed person, the condition itself tends to drive others away. Depressives often suffer from related physical ailments and frequently consult a physician for headaches, or backaches, or stomachaches, but not for being depressed, which not uncommonly leads to a misdiagnosis of the primary condition. This was what almost occurred with me and a patient I will call "Richard."

Richard and His Wrist

Thirty-eight-year-old Richard, his wife, and their five-year-old daughter had just moved to town, needed to establish care with a family physician, and ultimately became my patients. When Richard first came to see me about wrist pain, he struck me as a pleasant sort of fellow, if somewhat mild and quiet. He'd recently been hired by the university as a technician who made adjustments on a certain specialized form of microscope and was the only person on campus who knew how to perform that particular job.

We initially decided the wrist pain was due to an overuse syndrome from the manner in which he performed certain tasks. The standard new-patient history and physical turned up no other major health concerns. When Richard returned for a follow-up visit a month later, he reported he'd made alterations in his work patterns and that consequently the wrist was improving. That seemed to be the end of that, and I didn't expect another visit from Richard in the near future.

Richard was back in my office about eight months later, this time accompanied by his wife, Jenny. Jenny started our discussion by telling me they were seeking help for Richard's ten-year bout of depression—which took me aback, since the idea of depression hadn't crossed my mind. Jenny went on to explain that Richard would go to work, come home, and immediately want to go to sleep. On weekends he slept as much as possible, explaining that his work was highly stressful and that he needed his rest. Jenny felt he'd withdrawn to the point that he was no longer functioning as a husband and father. At work, he was able to spend all day among his microscopes, barely interacting with other people and, outside of his job and his family, he seemed to have no friends or social life.

I began treating Richard with antidepressant medication. During the next three months, he and Jenny came back to see me several times to report on his progress—which, after the initial two weeks it took the drug to kick in, was amazing to both of them. Admitting how different he felt now, Richard said his only regret was not having had his depression diagnosed sooner.

Depression: A Clinical Definition

A commonly accepted myth about depression is that it amounts to a lack of willpower, that if the depressed person would only try harder to cheer up and snap out of it, she could get better on her own. Many people with depression have their suffering increased because of this myth—because seeking help, which is what they need to do to get better, is made to seem like a personal failure. I find it much more plausible and supportive to view depression as arising from a chemical imbalance in the brain.

Here's how a nondepressed brain works. One brain cell talks to its neighbors by means of molecules called neurotransmitters, which basically carry messages across the gaps between the cells. In order for your brain to work properly, you must have a certain level of these neurotransmitter molecules in the spaces between the cells. The level of these molecules, in turn, depends on two processes that go on in the brain cells. The neurotransmitter molecules are manufactured, and then they are reabsorbed back into the cells. A nice balance between the manufacturing process and the reabsorption (or re-uptake) process assures the right amount of neurotransmitters in the spaces between the cells.

In contrast, with depression, the manufacturing process continues, but, for some mysterious reason, the re-uptake process is turned way too high, like a huge vacuum cleaner which sucks up all the neurotransmitters from the space between the brain cells. When one cell wants to talk to the cell next to it, no one's available to carry the message. This explains why the depressed person not only feels blue, but also has too little energy for turning thought into action. When you watch a severely depressed person talk or move, it's like watching a videotape in slow motion.

I hope the preceding explanation has made the point that the depressed person is not to blame for the social isolation in which he might find himself. Giving a depressive the list of guidelines we reviewed in the previous section would simply not help, since she needs to deal with social isolation in a way that takes her disease fully into account.

Conventional medicine invokes the neurotransmitter theory only to claim that, since depression is a chemical disease, it should have an exclusively chemical cure—namely, antidepression medication. It's my own belief as a family physician that these medications do in fact work, and in some cases work extremely well. We already saw that there's a contrary school of thought, which holds that antidepressants are really no more than fancy placebos, or that a goodly portion of the improvement they produce is actually attributable to a placebo response. What I object to as a family physician is not the use of antidepressants, but rather the idea that only these drugs are effective in relieving depression. I strongly believe that counseling, preferably in tandem with medication, is extremely helpful for cases of mild to moderate depression. Lifestyle changes, especially exercise, can also be very helpful. But you yourself have a critical role to play in getting better.

It's Up to You

Let me repeat: My message to the depressed person is that, while you are not to blame for your depression (or for the loneliness that goes along with it), you *can* in fact play a positive role in doing something about it. Your inner pharmacy is a potentially powerful ally—especially when depression is severe and you enlist help from the outer pharmacy, too. I would also recommend talking as soon as possible with a physician or other qualified healer, because part of the nature of the disease is that depressives don't realize how seriously ill they have become.

The most crucial aspect of handling depression, though, will be the importance of taking small steps rather than attempting to tackle the whole problem at once.

We previously used the example of picking up the phone to call your cousin whom you've been meaning to contact for the last couple of years. For most of us who aren't depressed, this fairly simple step is pretty intimidating. Asking a depressive with depleted neurotransmitters to make this call might seem tantamount to demanding she call the U.N. General Assembly into emergency session. A depressed person's taking a very tiny step toward greater social involvement—even getting out of the house for half an hour to go to the store—needs to be acknowledged as a major proactive measure in managing her own health. The goal is to have each tiny step lead to another tiny step.

Social Support Groups

There are a great many groups, as we've noted, through which you can become involved in meaningful social connections. Joining any one of them could be an extremely positive experience for someone whose illness has led to social isolation. The idea that it's a good thing for you to get your mind off your troubles may sound trite and old-fashioned, but it contains a substantial grain of truth. For some people who have been struggling with a severe, chronic illness for years, just being reminded that there's a whole world outside of the illness can be a step on the road to healing. Take this anecdote.

Granny Q's Kids

The nursing home was located in a white suburb, and the residents and staff were predominantly white. When four tall black teenagers strode into the lobby one afternoon, some of the staff started thinking stereotypical things and were prepared to retreat in fear. The four young men were pretty tight-lipped as they demanded to see "Granny Quentin."

Eventually the staff figured out that they meant Mrs. Quentin in room 17B, and went with some trepidation to tell her about her visitors. Mrs. Quentin, to their surprise, broke out in a huge grin. When the five of them met, it seemed like a family reunion.

The young men, it turned out, simply wanted to meet the woman who called them daily on the phone and helped them with their asthma. "There's not a one of us that has been in the hospital with an asthma attack for the past year," one of the boys later told a nurse. "And we've been maybe twice to the ER among the four of us. Before Granny Q, it was practically once a month."

The nursing home staff knew that Mrs. Quentin had been talking a lot more on the phone for the past year; but few of them knew she'd signed up for a senior volunteer program to help kids with asthma. The plan was to call in the morning before school, make sure they had used their peak flow meters, which measure early signs of breathing problems in time to start extra treatment if needed, and generally see how they were doing.

The organizers of the volunteer program reported that the kids showed an 80 percent drop in hospital days and half as many ER visits after the program got going. What about the elderly volunteers, most of whom were homebound or living in a residential care facility? A study of the volunteers revealed a marked reduction in depressive symptoms, and major improvements in meaning and well-being.

Musing about her own experience with the program, Mrs. Quentin said, "I used to wake up each morning wondering if that would finally be the day I was going to die. Now I wake up each morning and wonder how my kids are doing."

The bottom line is that group support works. If you want your group experience to be successful, there's a basic warning of which you should be aware.

Going with the Flow

When you join the group, you need to join the group. Any group exists for a specific reason; you need to accept that reason and adopt it as your own. If the group is a pottery class, its reason is to learn how to make pottery. If it's a Bible study group, it's to read and discuss the Bible. As much as you wish you could find a group that would listen to you talk about your illness and then offer you sympathy and compassion, that's not the main reason why the group exists. As time goes by, the others will probably listen to you, offer you emotional support, and make you feel like you belong—but they will do this precisely to the extent that they sense you are really one of them. Acting as if you intend to hijack the group for your own personal agenda is a sure way to turn off those who might otherwise be quite happy to be at your side.

In the rest of this section I want to talk about one special form of social support group: the ones created for the purpose of addressing the needs of people with a particular illness.

Disease-Focused Groups

This sort of group offers special benefits for you and your inner pharmacy, and also creates the risk for some unique pitfalls. First, an illustrative case study:

Group Therapy for Metastatic Breast Cancer

In the late 1970s, Dr. David Spiegel and a team of colleagues at Stanford University designed a special group treatment for women with breast cancer that had already spread to other parts of their body. They also studied a control arm, which did not take part in the group treatment. The groups, which met weekly for a year, had a number of features:

- They were led by a trained mental health worker in tandem with a therapist who herself had breast cancer.
- Women in the group were encouraged to discuss how to cope with cancer.
- The women were taught a self-hypnosis strategy to help them deal with pain.
- The groups encouraged discussion of feelings about cancer and the effect it had on their lives.

- Members formed strong bonds with each other to combat social isolation.
- Members worked with each other to assist everyone in becoming more assertive with their doctors.
- One focus of the discussion was how to extract meaning from the tragedy of breast cancer.
- The leaders encouraged the women to face losses squarely and go through the grieving process rather than to avoid or deny death and loss. One group held a meeting at the home of a member who was dying.

Dr. Spiegel and his colleagues were quite clear on one conclusion. They took a dim view of claims made by others that this kind of psychological-social intervention could actually extend life. They never told group members they expected them to live longer. After the group had ended, the research team kept track of the patients for a ten-year follow-up period. What the investigators hoped to be able to show was that their treatment program greatly improved the women's quality of life but had no effect on length of life.

Dr. Spiegel and his colleagues were quite surprised with their ten-year follow-up data. They were correct about one thing: The women reported improved quality of life compared to the control women who had not had the group sessions. But the group-treated women also lived longer. Indeed, they lived from fifteen to eighteen months longer on average, depending on exactly from which point you measured survival. After ten years, three of the treated women were still alive compared to none of the control subjects.

We can run down the list of issues addressed in Dr. Spiegel's group sessions and see much of what we have been talking about in previous chapters: taking more control, feeling cared for, and looking for positive meaning in illness. One key element of the meaning model is feeling you're surrounded by a group of people who demonstrate care and concern for you. And so it seems quite obvious. If you suffer from any sort of chronic disease, joining a social support group for persons with your illness will likely stimulate your inner pharmacy.

The additional advantage of such a social support group lies in the power of your story to shape how you cope with illness. Your task is to construct a story with the best possible outcome, in terms of making sense of the illness within the context of your life, and pointing you in the direction of getting on with your life and pursuing your most cherished goals despite the detour or interference the illness represents. Strong-willed and creative people could probably be hermits on a desert island and still manage to do this story work. For most of us, framing the stories of our lives, and of our illnesses, requires a lot of trying-out and trying-on. We need to bounce half-formed ideas of the story off others to see how they react. And we need to hear others tell similar stories, so that we get new ideas which we can incorporate into our own narratives. A social support group is the ideal story workshop for people trying to make sense of and come to terms with a serious chronic illness.

All these advantages exist merely with the idea of social support. Various illness support groups provide additional benefits as well. If, as happened with Dr. Spiegel's group, the leader is an experienced psychotherapist, members can learn such highly useful healing skills as relaxation and self-hypnosis, which encourage the placebo response and trigger the inner pharmacy. These groups are often great sources of information about the illness, from expert group leaders and from the members sharing among themselves the latest ideas they've gotten from the Internet or elsewhere. And for such conditions as addictions, the group itself may be the major form of treatment.

Joining a social support group might seem like a no-lose proposition. Unfortunately, it's not quite that easy. Caroline Myss reflecting on why some people seem to resist healing, developed the concept of "woundology." Woundology occurs when a basically healthy process goes astray. The healthy process is, first, seeking social support when one is ill; and second, realizing that if one has such deeply buried psychic wounds as having been brought up in an abusive or seriously dysfunctional family, then getting more in touch with those wounds and talking about them in a supportive environment is a first important step toward healing.

What, then, could go astray? The path to real healing moves beyond getting in touch with and talking about one's wounds. Eventually you have to tell (and live) a story of your life that allows you to get beyond the limitations the wounds impose, so that you are living your life, and not letting the wounds live your life for you. "Getting in touch" establishes the jumping-off place of the story; we cannot allow it to become the end of the story.

Lurking in the background can be the two powerful forces we've mentioned earlier: fear of loss of identity and fear of loneliness. When the group as a whole starts to reinforce and multiply these feelings, then they can be almost impossible to resist. The result can be a "social support group" that is supporting all of its members in staying wounded rather than in being healed.

So just how can you assess a social support group for chronic illness to see if it's a plus or a minus for you? Here are some questions that may help.

Finding a Group You Can Heal With

How long have most people been in the group? You have to be careful here. First, different groups have different goals, and some take much longer than others to accomplish. Programs like Alcoholics Anonymous may of necessity be lifelong. Second, individuals take different periods of time to get the same task done. In any group, there will be a few people who seem to have been around since day one, yet are healing at their own pace. If you figure on average how long it should take to accomplish the group's main goals, then discover most members have been in the group much longer than that, it may be a sign that the group is stuck with its wounds and not really making much healing progress.

How does the group treat incoming and outgoing members? A healthy group will be sad to see a member leave, but at the same time happy that the member has made progress and is able to move on. A new member will disrupt things for a while during an inevitable period of adjustment, but will still be welcomed as a person in need of the group's care. If the group seems to have great difficulty letting go of a "graduate," or seems to have a lot of problems accepting a new member, then you might detect a level of stagnation which wouldn't be helpful for you.

How does the group handle differences in coping style? Normal human beings, faced with a major challenge like chronic illness, don't all deal with it in the same way. Putting an illness experience into the context of your life, and making it meaningful within your life story, requires that it fit your life and your story, not someone else's. A group that will help you heal can deal with this. They'll listen carefully and make useful, sensitive, and pertinent comments, as long as you are willing to do the same with the other members' stories.

The sort of group you want to avoid, by contrast, has one script which all members are supposed to read from at each meeting. Members seem so fragile that they can cope only by being sure that every other member of the group is coping in exactly the same way. If someone else is handling things a little differently, fear is raised that one person's way might be "wrong," and for such a fragile group, that's far too scary a thought. If you find the price of acceptance is buying into the group version of the right story of this particular illness, think about whether you should be looking elsewhere for social support.

How well do group members listen? Members have to listen carefully to catch the precise variations in each person's style and story. You cannot listen with half an ear, confident that you already know what's being related. It's natural that people struggling with a serious illness will be somewhat self-absorbed, and will have bad days when they seem unable to listen to others since they're preoccupied with their own problems. Over time, you should find that others are capable of listening to what every person is saying. A group in which people simply wait in line to speak but don't take the trouble to listen is not going to help you much with the story work that is such a critical part of creating meaning.

In this and the previous chapter, we've looked at two ways to alter the meaning of one's experience with illness: story work and social connections. While all aspects of positive meaning help to turn on the inner pharmacy, the notion of taking control, or mastery, is an especially important goal. In the next chapter, we will look at additional ways in which taking greater control over the illness and its treatment can lead to an enhanced placebo response from the inner pharmacy.

FIFTEEN

Taking Charge of Your Own Health

"It would be more satisfying to me, it would allow me to feel I owned my illness, if my urologist were to say, 'You know, you've worked this prostate of yours pretty hard. It looks like a worn-out baseball.' Nobody wants an anonymous illness. I'd much rather think that I brought it on myself than that it was a mere accident of nature."

—Anatole Broyard

You've surely heard the traditional AA saying, "Grant me the courage to change the things I can change, the patience to endure the things I cannot change, and the wisdom to know the difference." Although it may have become overly familiar, the adage contains one of the most essential lessons for learning to be as healthy as you can. Now let's turn it around so its message is negative: There are two things that are almost sure to make you feel, and to be, less healthy: failing to do what you can to become healthier on a day-to-day basis, and worrying about things over which you actually have no control. It's astonishing how much valuable energy we waste doing both.

Once you tell yourself a healing story, and realize it could have a happy and meaningful ending, what must you do day by day to live it out? And what does taking charge of your health look like?

Components of Health Self-Management

Here's an anecdote to start off our discussion.

Women's Complaints

Dr. Kirsti Malterud is a family physician practicing on the coast of Norway. Some years ago, she became interested in a group of female patients with symptoms in the lower abdomen or pelvis—what her colleagues term "women's complaints." The patients had seen a number of gynecologists and family practitioners (usually male) and received a variety of diagnoses and treatments, none of which provided relief. One by one, all the other doctors had thrown up their hands. If they were polite, they said there was nothing more they could do. If they weren't, they would come flat out and declare, "There's nothing wrong with you. It's all in your head." Eventually, these women made their way to Dr. Malterud, perhaps hoping that as a woman, she would sympathize with them.

Wondering if the way she communicated with the women during office visits might make a difference in their health, Dr. Malterud experimented with several different approaches. Finally she devised a set of questions which she routinely asked whenever she saw one of the women. Over time, Malterud discovered that simply asking these questions seemed to produce positive health changes in her patients; their symptoms gradually subsided, and they were able to resume their normal lives.

A key question Dr. Malterud made a point of asking was, "And what do you think you should do about the problem [that brought you in to see me today]?" As it turned out, none of the women's other doctors had asked such a question, preferring "Here's what you should do," or the aforementioned "There's nothing we can do." It occurred to Dr. Malterud that, in all their previous medical care, the women had been repeatedly receiving the message, "You are totally helpless in managing your problem and your life." Simply suggesting they could perhaps do something and that their ideas about what it should be were worth listening to seemed to produce a major healing effect.

The placebo response is *one* component of wellness and healing; your health—and your health story—involve many features beside it, including nutrition, exercise, medicines, or herbal remedies, which commonly come first, with the placebo response arriving as a supplement.

For instance, you review the story of your struggle with some chronic illness (let's say, diabetes) now that you've given it a better ending. You decide that getting more exercise is a major element of that new narrative. So you work out a plan to fit exercise into your schedule, choose a type of exercise you really enjoy, and locate a gym that's accessible and convenient. Then you proceed actually to carry out your plan.

In this example, your health and your control over the diabetes is clearly going to improve because of your new exercise program. I wouldn't consider that improvement to be a placebo response. In addition, there is the positive mental effect of having successfully taken charge of a portion of your life, and of the enhanced sense of being in control that results from it. This mental effect, as we saw in the earlier chapters, can send a prescription to the body's inner pharmacy, adding extra power to what the body is already using to fight the diabetes. So the total healing power unleashed by the exercise program is comprised of the healthy effects of exercise itself plus the placebo response.

The case study that follows provides another clue to how feeling more in charge can lead to better health.

Remembering to Take Your Placebo Every Day

Back in the 1980s, a group of investigators, who called themselves the Coronary Drug Project Research Group, were attempting to prevent deaths from heart attack by lowering cholesterol and other lipid (fatty) substances in the bloodstream. All 8,341 patients in their study, which was being conducted simultaneously at fifty-three medical centers around the country, were advised to follow a low-saturated-fat diet and to exercise. In randomized double-blind fashion, some subjects were also receiving a lipid-lowering drug called clofibrate, while others were getting a placebo.

As part of the research, pill counts were conducted to see if people were taking the medication, a procedure that would become important when the final data were analyzed. Ultimately, the investigators compared the mortality rates in those who took their clofibrate as prescribed and those who frequently forgot to take it. And indeed a statistically significant difference emerged. There was a substantially higher death rate among poor pill-takers than among patients who, as doctors say, were compliant. So it would seem at first that clofibrate must be truly effective in preventing deaths from heart attack.

Of course that was not the whole story. When the investigators next looked at the figures for the placebo arm, they found the same thing: Those who were very compliant with taking their placebos had a lower death rate than those who often forgot to take them. In the end, the study showed no significant difference in heart attacks and deaths between the clofibrate and the placebo groups.

Since that initial study, a number of other large-scale trials, many of them also dealing with drugs for heart disease, have shown the same phenomenon. High-compliance patients do better than low-compliance patients, whether they are taking the drug or the placebo.

Skeptics about the placebo response point to this sort of difference as another reason to deny that the placebo response is real. Remember, they suggest that high-compliance patients do better in these studies because they take better care of their health and follow doctors' orders to the letter. A careful review of a number of studies suggests that differences in health behavior alone cannot explain the entire effect of compliance. Though we're not yet completely sure what is happening in these studies, one possible explanation is that people who remember to take all their pills may feel more in charge, and this mental boost may help to stimulate their inner pharmacies.

Give Yourself Credit

One often-forgotten step in unleashing your mental power for enhanced health is to think consciously about it. Don't just do it; be aware of the fact that you're doing it. Consider the exercise-diabetes example we just mentioned. Here, you went through three different levels of taking charge:

- Retelling the story of the diabetes so that it had a better ending.
- Planning to start a regular exercise program.
- Actually doing the exercise every day.

If you're like most of us, it's probably difficult for you to change deep-set habits. Maybe you did a great job on the first two levels, but you're really struggling with the third one. What do you tell yourself? Many people would say, "I'm a failure; I need to exercise for my diabetes and I just can't seem to do it." The better answer is, "I have taken charge at two of the three levels; now I just have to work harder to gain mastery at the third level."

Since we're talking about mind and meaning, it's wise to remember that your attitude toward what you're doing is just as important as what you do. So give yourself full credit for whatever you are taking charge of, and start to see yourself more as a person who is taking charge and less as a person to whom unhealthy things just happen. This take-charge attitude will help stoke up your inner pharmacy; and it will also build your momentum, giving you more motivation and will-power to tackle what still remains to be done.

What if feeling in charge is especially hard for you? To try to get yourself over the hump, you can employ a trick some counselors use very effectively.

Keeping Score: The Mastery Percentage

Here's the trick. Begin by asking yourself "To what extent is *my disease* running my life and how much am *I* running my life?" Then assign a percentage score to both questions and see how you feel about your answers.

Suppose you're a person with diabetes who says, "I think that my diabetes is 15 percent in charge of my life and I am in charge of the other 85 percent." This could be an acceptable percentage, because you have to share your life to some extent with a disease like diabetes; you can't simply ignore it. Giving diabetes *some* control over your life actually makes you healthier because it makes you take care both of it and of yourself. But perhaps you decide, "I feel as if the diabetes is running 70 percent of my life and I am 30 percent in charge." That sounds like a much more serious imbalance: You'll probably feel and function a lot healthier if the mastery percentage is increased.

The question becomes: "When I think back on whatever small, temporary successes I've had in taking control of my life away from the disease, which things have worked best for me at different times?" Carefully considering this issue will almost always produce a list of practical, realistic steps. For instance, it's possible that last week, the time you felt most in control was when you ate that salad at lunch that you really liked. It happened to have been a healthy thing for you to eat; but at the time, you told yourself that you were eating it because it tasted good and not because your diabetes "made" you.

Next you ask yourself, "Now that I know what has worked some of the time to enhance my taking charge of my own life, how can I start doing more of these things every day?" The answer will produce a plan for building up your mastery percentage. In our example, this might prompt you to make a list of foods which you really enjoy eating and which also happen to be healthy for a person with diabetes, and promise yourself that you'll eat more foods from this "win-win" list.

Once you've got your plan, set a time each week to review the events of the past seven days and write down the new percentage score. Then, every month or two, look back over the recent weeks' scores and see what headway you're making.

Let's say you first recorded a 70/30 split in favor of the diabetes; after working to improve the split for a month, you record a new percentage of 60/40—a big step in the right direction. You then review the past month and ask yourself, "What worked best?" Now you can refine your take-charge plan to include even more of what's working, magnifying the chance that by the following month, your mastery percentage will be even higher.

Keeping score of the mastery percentage gets to the heart of the issue of whether or not you feel in control of your own health. Most importantly, it ties your take-charge attitude to practical steps: As you're gaining greater mastery over your own life, you start to *feel* more in charge even before the practical activity has fully paid off in terms of daily function. It's almost as if you got the placebo response before you even swallowed the pill; yet you still get to swallow it and reap its benefits later on. The anecdote below is a perfect example of the mastery percentage in action.

Wesley's Migraines

Do you remember the story of Hank's battling his migraines in chapter 13? It turned out that Hank was not the only chronic migraine sufferer I treated whose pain could be controlled only with high doses of narcotics. There was "Wesley," who also became my patient.

Wesley was a thirty-year-old gay man in a committed long-term relationship. Like Hank, he could fill a notebook with a list of all the physicians, evaluations, and treatments that had failed him. Unlike Hank, Wesley could count only on perhaps one day a week when he didn't have a headache. He'd sustained a severe head injury at about age twenty, which led me to suspect he suffered from a mixed type of headache that was especially resistant to treatment. Besides the narcotics and muscle relaxants I continued to prescribe for him in staggering doses every month, Wesley was trying a series of such alternative therapies as acupuncture, which seemed promising at first but eventually had little overall impact on the headaches.

When I suggested we work on the meaning of these headaches in his life as our best way of weaning him off the narcotics, Wesley immediately agreed. I ran into an unexpected problem when I urged him to start keeping a journal of every facet of his headaches he could think of on a daily or weekly basis. He consented, but several months went by with no journal appearing in my office. This made me wonder about the influence of something from his past. Finally, I put him on the spot and gently goaded him into telling me about his childhood.

Based on his own account, Wesley seemed to have an emotionally abusive mother. Although he was extremely intelligent, he didn't remember ever having earned praise from her. On the contrary, in her eyes he was a disappointment and a failure. Once he opened up to me, the source of his difficulty in writing the journal soon emerged.

Wesley had been repeatedly told by his mother that his writing was a disgrace: His grammar was awful, his spelling atrocious, his handwriting illegible. To this day, he couldn't put pen or pencil to paper without a scolding Mom appearing in his imagination to call him more names.

I had hopes at this point that perhaps I'd gotten to the secret of Wesley's headaches. He began to see a counselor and over time was able to get help with his feelings of worthlessness. He was even able to start writing some journal entries for me to discuss with him. But I was disappointed to see that these improvements in his psychological state didn't in the least affect his headaches.

Though I didn't give up on the journal, I searched for some other means to get at the headache problem. At last, I decided to give the mastery percentage a trial, with Wesley initially scoring 80 percent for the migraine's control of his life and 20 percent for himself. He felt especially guilty about this because of his partner. They would often go on trips, planning to have fun, yet Wesley inevitably ended up curled in a fetal position on a hotel bed, ruining both their vacations. At home, his inability to do much cooking and housework also placed extra burdens on his partner.

I told Wesley that each month I'd be asking him for the mastery percentage; meanwhile he was to devise a strategy which might increase the amount of control he had over his life.

During the next year or so, some small victories occurred. Despite his almost daily migraines and all the medication, Wesley decided to do more of the housework, especially on headache-free days. He was pleased to tell me that the mastery percentage had shifted somewhat away from the disease to perhaps 75/25.

The next victory came through the journal, which he worked on from time to time; eventually, he showed me two surprising entries. In one, he recalled he'd once held a job in the art field and been quite successful at it. For the first time in years, he was starting to contemplate getting back into the art work which he loved. In the other entry, he listed political and social causes about which he felt keenly, and offered the hope that he could try to make the world better for other people, not just for himself. He was beginning to create the glimmerings of a better life story in which the headaches didn't keep him from his goals.

The third victory, according to Wesley, was life-altering. As he worked with his counselor on childhood issues, he had a sudden realization: His mother treated him the way she did not because of him, but because of herself. It was the warped way she saw the world, shaped in turn by the warped way that she herself had been raised, that led her to be condemning and abusive to him. Wesley must have heard that message over and over from doctors and counselors, but only now was he finally receiving and fully internalizing it. He really did feel as if his life had turned around.

Although he had never told me this before, Wesley customarily stayed in bed as long as he could in the morning, often blaming the headaches when actually he simply found the world an unpleasant place. After his realization about his mother, he began getting up early and doing even more around the house. For the first time since he could remember, the world seemed inviting. Any expert reading this would probably take me to task for failing to diagnose and treat Wesley's long-term depression; but antidepressants were among the long list of medications that had previously been tried with no effect on him.

Wesley's basic relationship with his mother remained unchanged; he still saw her as a very unpleasant woman whom he tried to avoid as much as possible, which seemed wise in terms of his getting better. After all, who needs negative reinforcement, especially from so formative a figure in your life? His mastery percentage shifted again, awarding Wesley 40 percent and the headaches 60 percent. Given the snail's pace at which we'd been moving, this shift seemed a major step forward.

I'm rather reluctant at this time to make any predictions about where we'll eventually get with Wesley's treatment. His headaches are among the most severe I have ever tried to manage. But I have no doubt about two things. First, where we have seen any progress at all, it has come through activities or events that seemed to alter what the headaches meant to him. And secondly, one single activity, management scoring, genuinely seemed to help Wesley be more in control of various aspects of his own life and his own care.

"Guaranteed Success"—Taking Small Steps

RIDDLE: How do you eat an elephant?

ANSWER: One bite at a time.

It seems to me that the major reason many people aren't taking reasonable charge of their own health is because they get themselves into a double bind. They feel they have only two choices: Swallow the elephant whole by trying to tackle the entire problem right away; or do nothing and let the sickness or threat of it control them. Because swallowing the elephant whole is an impossible task, the only remaining alternative is permanent victimhood.

Once again let's steal a trick from good counselors, who can help us eventually to change very deeply rooted patterns of thinking and behavior by showing us how to take it one small step at a time. Often, the first practical action in managing an aspect of your illness or health is to break it down into small pieces so that you can start working with a feasible portion of the problem. In fact, the goal of such a process is termed "guaranteed success."

When you begin to take charge, your first thought might be that unless you really get going full bore, and try to gobble this huge elephant, you won't get anywhere and your health will worsen. One possible result is that you are so intimidated by the huge goal that you end up doing nothing at all. The other possible result is trying something big the first time around—like trying to stop smoking, give up coffee, lose weight, and cut down on your drinking all at the same time. Usually such an attitude leads to a further result, which is that your attempt doesn't succeed; and that leads to a third result: your becoming so demoralized by your "failure" that you never make another attempt.

But it need not be this way.

Helping Preston Find a Job

"Preston" is now my patient, but this event happened some years ago, when he was being cared for by a partner in my practice. At the time, Preston had been off work for several years, after an accident that left him with chronic, severe mid-back pain. He was getting care from a pain clinic, which was set up as a team effort and held monthly staff meetings to see how each patient was progressing.

After a while, Preston was doing much better in terms of physical pain and function. Indeed, it seemed he would actually beat the odds and soon be back at work; at the team meetings, the psychologist and vocational rehabilitation counselor always mentioned that Preston was planning to start job-hunting soon. But months and months went by, with Preston no closer to getting a job.

Then something dramatic happened. The vocational rehabilitation counselor got Preston into a special program called a "job club." What this "club" did was break down the task of job hunting into the smallest possible steps: first you polish up your résumé; then you look in the want ads; next you circle the ads that describe jobs that you could do or might want to do; then you call the numbers; and so on.

Somehow, after dealing for so many years with his back pain, and the depression and anxiety that accompanied it, Preston could not face the task of job hunting so long as it loomed above him as one single, huge challenge. All that was needed to get him going was the apparently simple-minded business of taking small steps. Two months after starting with the job club, Preston was employed full time.

Thus, the ideal plan is to select a small, simple step initially so you can almost be guaranteed you'll succeed. As you follow up with later steps, add only a small bit to the complexity or difficulty of what you are asking of yourself. If, when you get to a later step and fall flat on your face, it only means you need to back off and keep things simpler or easier for a while longer. The goal of this process is to cement in your mind the experience of succeeding as early as possible. This alters your attitude to coping successfully with your health problems, which in turn stimulates the inner pharmacy, making it more likely you'll succeed at later steps even though they get progressively harder.

You might of course ask, "If all I take at the beginning is little baby steps, doesn't that mean I'll never make it far enough to tackle the really big things?" Physicians who do a lot of lifestyle counseling know that this is almost never the problem. Rather, patients are more likely to fail in the end because they start out like gangbusters, then find they can't keep up the pace, and consequently drop out of the process after a week or a month or several months. It's the ability to stick it out over the long haul, not the ability to take a big stride right off the bat, that determines success or failure. So, for guaranteed success, you can almost never go wrong by starting with the small step.

Besides the attitudinal benefits of "guaranteed success," you'll also start to view the world differently. If you feel that the only way to take control of a health problem is to attack it all at once, then the world looks very threatening and scary. Once you redefine the problem as smaller steps in a long term process, what you now see when you look around is much more manageable. The thought more likely to cross your mind now is, "I can handle this." That certainly helps to firm up a take-charge attitude and dispel your feelings of victimization.

All this talk of small steps instead of big steps may seem pretty abstract. Here are some common examples of going for "guaranteed success," a few of which we've mentioned—but which definitely merit repeating:

- Addiction programs like Alcoholics Anonymous are now famous for their twelve step approach.

- When starting an exercise program, think first about carving out a safe, predictable time of day when you know that you can exercise;

and do that even if the actual amount of exercise is minimal. If you want to do sit-ups and you're in such bad shape that your body hurts after you do five, then do three or four. Once you can do three or four once each day, then add one extra sit-up per day for a while, or even just one every week.

- Changing your diet: Don't throw out all your old eating habits and start over completely. Set a goal to do something different at one meal or with one item of food, for example, changing to a low-fat salad dressing. Don't take any additional steps until you've gotten the low-fat salad dressing habit down firmly. Remember, start with the things that will be easiest to change and save the harder steps for later on, after your initial success.

- "One day at a time" is always a good maxim to follow when change seems overwhelming. Stop yourself from thinking too far into the future and just plan to do whatever needs to be accomplished to succeed today.

- When failure happens—you're human, so it will—resist the temptation to make global judgments of guilt and blame ("Oh no! I blew it!"). First, tell yourself that no one starts out to do something difficult and worthwhile without stumbling along the way. Second, remind yourself that a so-called failure is not really a failure but a learning opportunity: What do you now know about what works and what doesn't that you didn't know before? How can you use this new knowledge to help achieve greater or more consistent success in the future? For instance, if you've been smoke-free for several weeks, and then light up a cigarette when you go with your friends to a certain bar, you'll come to realize that this bar (or maybe those friends) is bad news for your good-health efforts.

Climbing Back on the Wagon

If you're not making the progress you'd hoped for with small steps, it helps to reexamine the basic starting point. Make sure that what you set out to manage is an aspect of your health over which you actually have control. If you made a mistake and tried to change something over which you have no control, then it's obvious why you didn't succeed. If you're in doubt about this, you may need to consult with your physician or other healer.

To give just one example, some people with adult-type diabetes have levels of sugar in the bloodstream that naturally pop up and down for no apparent reason all day long. These people may have rather high blood sugars at certain times each day, even when their diabetes overall is well-controlled with diet, exercise, medicines, and perhaps insulin shots. I have seen diabetic patients who compulsively check their blood sugar levels with home monitoring machines six or eight times each day, keep a record of all the numbers, and come to the physician shaking their heads woefully about the continued high readings. They may keep doing this when other tests, which more accurately reflect the long term control of the diabetic disease process, actually show that things are improving.

These particular patients need to calm down and realize that, though they can control their diet, their exercise, and their taking their medicines—and by doing this, lower the chance that they will get later complications of diabetes—they simply are not going to be able to control their blood sugar from minute to minute. They should put their little monitoring machines in the drawer and forget about them. In the majority of patients, of course, the regular monitoring of their blood sugar is a vital part of taking control; so this example refers only to a special group of diabetics who have discussed this thoroughly with their physicians.

Practice for Success

The following story, which comes from Caroline Myss, makes an important point that can be useful for a variety of illnesses.

Julio's "Faking It"

Julio, who had been going in and out of depression for a long time, probably suffered from seasonal affective disorder; he always seemed to bottom out during the winter. When in the middle of one of these states, he would spend most of his time sitting in front of the TV with a blank stare. His wife tried to help him as much as possible, suggesting a variety of distracting activities, but finally tired of his lack of response—"she hit the ceiling" was how Julio later put it.

She told him he could sit around and be depressed if he wanted to, but she was sick of having his anchor pulling her down as well. From now on, she announced, she was going to go out and enjoy life even if he wouldn't. When she came home from frequent evenings out with friends, she always made it a point to tell Julio what a good time she'd had. Next she moved out of their bedroom, claiming Julio was just too boring to be around, and that if she didn't avoid him, she'd be getting depressed herself.

During a healing workshop he attended sometime later, Julio described what happened subsequently:

"I was hurt at first by her remarks, and then I got scared. I couldn't stand the thought of losing her, so I just made the decision to snap out of it, even if I had to fake the appearance of being out of my depression. I started to force myself to go out with her and do things together. It was very, very difficult at first, because I was still so depressed. It felt artificial to act as though I weren't depressed, but I didn't have any choice.

"In the long run, though, my determination actually healed my condition, because I began to feel that I was in charge of my moods instead of my depression controlling me. Now when I feel the mood swing coming on, I also feel that I have a choice to fight back. And I have my wife to thank for it."

Now for the warning: Julio's wife's "treatment" of depression falls clearly under the *Don't try this at home!* category. In a severe depression this could easily backfire. Indeed the wife was fortunate that her strategy didn't cause Julio to commit suicide.

To urge the depressed person to "snap out of it" ignores the fact that he simply lacks the adequate brain chemistry to take effective action for himself. If he could snap out of it, he wouldn't have the disease called depression. In retrospect, Julio was lucky to suffer from only a chemically mild case of the disease, making it possible for his wife to evoke a positive, self-healing reaction in him.

Now that we've established how not to treat depression most of the time, let's take advantage of our 20/20 hindsight in Julio's case. Since we know that something did work, let's analyze what it was. It seems significant that Julio improved as a result of feeling that he was finally taking charge of his life and wresting control away from his illness. A particularly important discovery in his story was the role of "faking it." We are often far too harsh on such so-called pretense, not realizing that what we derisively call faking may actually be trying.

All of us have to try on a complex action before we can succeed at it. If we stopped trying right away because the behavior felt funny or insincere—which we would expect, because it takes a long time for any new behavior pattern to become smoothly part of ourselves and to feel like we own it—then we'd give up far too soon and never gain the advantage of this critical change for the better.

So the general lesson which I recommend we take away from Julio's atypical case of depression is this*:* How important it is to try a new, healthier pattern of behavior, even when initially it feels phony or insincere. After all, the important point for your sincerity and personal integrity is not what you are doing this minute, but what you aim to do with your life. If you are disgusted with your habitual smoking and sincere in your goal to quit, then trying on nonsmoking behaviors is not really being phony or hypocritical.

Of course it feels odd, since behaving in a way that is different from your long-ingrained patterns always does for a while. But the odd feeling is a very poor indicator of the real you. You have already determined that the real you is going to be the nonsmoking you. Trying harder to be that sort of person, even in the small steps that you have to use at first in order to be sure that you succeed, is a positive expression of the real, healthier you.

We imagine in Julio's case that his trying on nondepressed behavior may have been a part of the trigger for his inner pharmacy to cause his brain to make more of the missing neurotransmitters, steering him toward the eventual complete recovery from depression. In your own case, it's important not to let the strangeness of new, healthier patterns of behavior cause you to stop too quickly. It may take a little while before your inner pharmacy gets the full message from your new way of acting.

In the last few chapters we've talked about turning on your inner pharmacy by paying more attention to meaning and mastery. Here and there, we found that it's better to rely on the help of professional practitioners. Are there special ways of selecting those practitioners who are most likely to work in an effective partnership with you, and with your inner pharmacy? We'll take up that question in the next chapter.

SIXTEEN

Sustaining a Partnership: Sharing Control with Physicians and Other Healers

"[The physician Ralph Bloomfield Bonington is] . . . cheering, reassuring, healing by the mere incompatibility of disease or anxiety with his welcome presence. Even broken bones, it is said, have been known to heal at the sound of his voice; he is a born healer . . . "

—George Bernard Shaw, 1911

In the past few chapters we've looked at ways to get the most out of your inner pharmacy on your own. Now we will talk about how to boost your inner pharmacy when working together with a healer, either a physician or an alternative practitioner, with whom you can form a bond.

Choosing the Right Healer

Almost ninety years ago, the playwright George Bernard Shaw seemed aware of what makes some practitioners more proficient than others at turning on our inner pharmacies. In his 1911 play *The Doctor's Dilemma,* Shaw created the character Sir Ralph Bloomfield Bonington, M.D., whose healing prowess is celebrated in the quotation that opens this chapter. Shaw referred to Bonington as "a born healer," but in my experience, you don't have to be born a healer to become what I like to call "a healing sort of person." The necessary skills—which we'll be discussing later on—can be taught to aspiring physicians in medical school and residency.

Has contemporary medical science come up with hard evidence suggesting that the nature of your healer and of your mutual relationship actually makes a difference in getting better? Here's an illuminating and widely cited case study, carried out by British general practitioner Dr. K. B. Thomas.

The Power of Positive Talking

Dr. Thomas, like all general and family practitioners, saw many patients who complained of various symptoms but seemed to have no clear medical diagnosis. With no diagnosis, there was not a convincing reason to give them medical treatment. Dr. Thomas decided to see how two different actions affected their health: talking to them in a positive way; and giving them some form of treatment regardless.

Dr. Thomas selected two hundred such patients and randomly assigned them to four groups of fifty each. Half the patients got a positive message: "I know just what is wrong with you, and I'm confident that you'll be good as new in only a few days." Half got a negative message: "I really don't know what's the matter with you." Within each of these groups, half of each group received a prescription for a pill: The positive group was told that the pill would certainly make them better; the negative group was informed that the doctor was really not sure if the pill would help. The other half of each group got no prescription. The positive group was told that since the disease naturally got better in a few days, no medicine was needed; the negative group was told that no medicine could be given since the doctor had been unable to arrive at a diagnosis. The four groups of fifty were: positive-prescription; positive-no prescription; negative-prescription; negative-no prescription. The two prescription groups received a placebo in the form of extremely low doses of vitamin B_1.

On leaving the office, patients filled out questionnaires relating to how satisfactory they'd found the visit. Two weeks later they were mailed a card asking them if they'd improved and, if so, how long it had taken them to get better.

Dr. Thomas discovered after reviewing this data that taking the placebo prescription by itself made no difference in whether or not people reported getting better. Surprisingly, from our standpoint, no placebo effect as narrowly defined was seen in this study. But the positive vs. negative consultation made a great difference. The positive groups reported a 64 percent rate of getting better as compared to only a 39 percent improved rate in the negative groups. The positive groups also reported greater satisfaction with the visit.

It would be a godsend if all healers possessed an equally potent ability to turn on our inner pharmacies, but that's simply not the case. As we know, our inner pharmacies react positively to healing stimuli or healing messages, and healers differ markedly in their talent for sending these messages. Beyond that, people are individuals, and a healer who can send the best sort of message to one person may not be able to do so with another patient. This applies even when the healer is expert at the technical details of his science or craft.

To take a simple example, imagine that your sixty-eight-year-old Aunt Agatha is somewhat old-fashioned and feels most cared for when the healer is highly directive: She has a strong belief in "doctor's orders" and expects to be told what to do. Now let's think of two physicians, one a more old-fashioned, very friendly but rather authoritative type, and the other more recently trained, hence educated in patient's rights, the need to explain things thoroughly, answer questions, and ask patients what sort of treatment they're looking for. Though both doctors may be equally able as technicians and scientists, the first physician will probably be much more effective in turning on Aunt Agatha's inner pharmacy. The case might be exactly the opposite with her forty-year-old daughter.

This example indicates that you might have to invest considerable time and energy before you locate the best healer to consult. Even consulting with your friends and neighbors will not necessarily work for you, unless you're convinced they require the same attributes in a healer that you do.

Of course, this doesn't mean selecting a healer is as random an act as a roll of the dice. We've seen what general factors give positive meaning to an illness experience and thus have the most powerful influence on the inner pharmacy. The meaning model provides us with a good list of qualities to seek in a healer.

I believe you will make a sensible and informed decision if you keep the following questions in mind:

Does this healer take the time to explain things? We've seen that a good explanation is one of the key elements of meaning which turns on the inner pharmacy, but it customarily requires considerable clinical time. There are several different ways in which a practitioner might make that needed time. One is to extend the total length of the visit to allow for a thorough explanation. The other is efficient use of time even within a short visit. For instance, a physician can be talking to you while also looking in your throat or feeling your neck for lymph nodes. Either way, he's sending you a signal that allowing time for thorough explanations is a high priority of his.

Suppose there isn't sufficient time for a full explanation without putting the healer way behind schedule. If so, she may suggest you reschedule soon to make sure the two of you have another chance to talk. At first, you may be resentful because a second visit means taking extra time off work, or paying an extra fee. If you want real quality in a healing relationship, you need to be willing to invest in it. The healer who suggests a return visit specifically to talk over a complicated issue shows you in the strongest possible way how much she values effective communication.

Does the healer tailor the explanation to your personal needs and abilities? Can you easily grasp the manner in which he explains things? Does he size you up, then choose an explanation to dovetail with your educational level and past experience? Or do you get the feeling that this healer has one stock explanation for each disease or treatment and plays the same tape for everyone who walks in the door?

Does the healer signal to you that questions are welcome? Unless you're comfortable asking questions, it's unlikely you'll get an explanation that satisfies you. Healers are not mind-readers. If you don't ask, they'll never know whether the explanation was sufficient or if they weren't being clear. Most of us are slightly (or more than slightly) intimidated by healers. We often feel rushed during a typical office visit. It's easy to say "uh-huh" to a healer and nod when you really haven't a clue about what she is telling you. This means that most healers have to do a little extra work to put us enough at ease so that our questions flow.

While time spent for the visit can be easily measured, the little signals indicating the healer's interest or disinterest are harder to detect. An obvious illustration of disinterest is the practitioner who seems to go into a doze, starts to fidget, or gets up and puts his hand on the doorknob whenever we ask a question. As I've suggested, the cues are often more subtle—for instance, small changes in eye contact or tone of voice—but we pick them up just the same. Ask yourself whether the attitude you pick up during a visit welcomes or discourages questions.

Does the healer seem to care about you as a person? We've seen that caring is the second major element of meaning which stimulates the inner pharmacy. Again, this is a highly intangible aspect of your relationship with your healer. But it's feelings and gut impressions, not hard data, that are going to turn on your inner pharmacy. So you need to trust your instincts.

Do you get the impression over time that your healer is concerned about who you are and what all this means to you as a person, and doesn't see you simply as the body that happens to have whatever bundle of symptoms you complain of? Does it seem to matter to the healer whether or not you get better, not just out of professional pride, but out of genuinely caring for you? Does the healer seem to want to hear about your job, your family, and your hobbies, as well as your symptoms? If you can answer "yes" to most or all of these questions, she is probably transmitting an aura of caring, which will go a long way toward improving your response to treatment.

When you leave the office, consider your global impression. Do you feel better than you did when you came in? Have you received *care?* Do you sense that the caregiver is a healing sort of person? Did you experience a warm and close, but fully professional, human contact with her?

Does the healer help you feel more in control? Control or mastery is the third important element of the meaning model. The ideal healer will help you gain the best sense of being in charge of your life and your illness. Exactly what this means in practice is also not always easy to decipher.

The healer who makes you feel as if you have to rush to his office every time you cough or sneeze is obviously not going to make you feel more in control. What about the practitioner who sits down beside you as you're experiencing crushing chest pains, which you both believe is probably a heart attack, lists a myriad of complicated treatment choices, then asks you to think them over and select a single option on the spot? I doubt you'd find such a situation any more satisfactory.

Just how much control you ought to feel over your life and illnesses, and the exact way that control is exercised, ought to vary depending on the seriousness and urgency of your health condition and on how capable you feel at the time of exercising control. For instance, if you are severely depressed, it's quite unlikely that you'll respond to any offer of control in a meaningful way. There are times in any long-term healing relationship when the best action a healer can take is to exert control for you, at least temporarily. This is true even though I feel as a general rule that your being more in control is, in the long run, the healthiest way to behave. So maybe we should restate this question as:

Does the healer make you feel like a real partner in controlling your health and illness? We'll see later on that, in measuring the quality of physician-patient relations, some experts have suggested sustained partnership as the preferred model. To me, a true partnership determines how much control is merited at any given time. Being treated as a true partner means that you'll get to make all the important decisions for yourself. Your partner will not dictate to you, but you'll never feel alone or abandoned when weighty decisions have to be made. Your partner will stand beside you, offering any advice or expertise that could assist you. For those occasional times when you feel overwhelmed by events, your partner will step in and take charge, intent on turning the reins back over to you as soon as you are capable of assuming them.

All of us go through periods in our lives when, for no apparent reason, we feel incapable of making choices and taking charge; or we're just feeling stubborn and don't want to. What does a partner do in such circumstances? The ideal partner will understand and won't blame you for what is after all a very human trait, but neither will he take things at face value and assume you really want to retreat into infantile helplessness as your primary way of dealing with the world. With kindness and encouragement, he'll subtly steer you back to taking charge of your own life, not so rapidly that you can't handle it, but rapidly enough to prod and push just a little when you need some gentle persuasion.

Does your healer seem to become more powerful as you become more powerful? This is an important aspect of being the true partner we just talked about, but it's initially hard to grasp. Let me begin by describing what it doesn't mean.

I'm definitely not talking about the practitioner who always needs to be right, and who seems threatened by any signal that you've wrested control away from him. Let's say such a practitioner suggests you modify your diet in a certain way to lose weight, and you find that by doing it differently, you can stick with the regimen more easily and lose even more weight. Instead of congratulating you on your creativity and motivation, this physician becomes annoyed because you didn't follow his advice and then launches into a detailed discussion of why his original advice would have produced more impressive results.

This practitioner seems to regard power as a win-lose game. If you seem a bit more powerful, that power had to come from someplace, and this practitioner fears that some of his own power must have been lost in order for you to have gotten it. He's less concerned with how much better you are than with hanging onto every last bit of his own superiority. This guy is probably exactly what your inner pharmacy doesn't need, and you and he should find opposite paths to travel as soon as possible.

The type of healer I recommend realizes that power can grow exponentially in an effective healing partnership. His goal is to make you healthier. As you become more empowered in managing your own health, he can do an even better job of achieving his goal. Thus, he too becomes more powerful. The result is a win-win power situation. In any case, the notion of a win-lose game of power is not reality, but a mental trap.

As you grow more self-reliant, the ideal healing partner seems to become more energized. He congratulates you on your empowerment, then uses his expertise to suggest new things you can do that you couldn't previously. Even if you have used your control to do something that is actually not beneficial to your health, the healer still congratulates you for your greater mastery, then calmly suggests a better method to use in controlling your healing.

Let's suppose that as you recover from knee surgery, you're doing a graded rehabilitation and exercise program, and you're so eager to be fit again that you initially overdo things and put too much stress on the knee. Some physicians might chew you out and tell you in no uncertain terms that you've placed your recovery in jeopardy. By contrast, the ideal partner orthopedist would praise you for your intense desire to heal, then steer you back to a moderate level of exercise, reassuring you that with time you'll be able to enhance it.

Does the healer have a sense of humor? You might think I have in mind the experience of the late Norman Cousins, who claimed to have recovered from a life-threatening illness mainly by watching old Marx Brothers movies and laughing his head off. Laughter may indeed be very good medicine and is probably a fine stimulus for the inner pharmacy, but I'm not about to recommend you select a healer because he's a great stand-up comic.

Rather, my idea is that the healer you seek has a complicated set of personal traits. This practitioner is highly self-confident, but not arrogant. He is an assertive, take-charge person but is also prepared to stand aside and allow you to be in control along with him. And, yes, it does seem as if we're asking him to be a seamless weave of contradictory traits we usually don't expect to find in one person.

I know such people exist, and that one important quality they share seems to allow them to display many traits at once: They don't take themselves too seriously. The healer who can best turn on your inner pharmacy is often appropriately humble and modest about the outer pharmacy. He isn't so full of himself that he thinks all healing in his general vicinity occurs due to his own greatness. And I'd suggest that the healer who doesn't take himself too seriously frequently comes equipped with a healthy sense of humor.

What about the rest of the office staff? Few healers today are able to work in a vacuum. Usually, your first contact with the office will *not* be directly with the healer. Sometimes an encounter with a member of the office staff can undo all the good that has been carefully built up over time in the partnership with the healer. Are the good attributes of the healer shared by those who work with him? If the physician is very warm and interested in you, but the receptionist is rude, and the nurse is cold and indifferent, how comfortable will you feel going there over time?

Think about the questions I posed quite carefully. You will have your own ideas about priorities. You may come to one item and say to yourself, "Yes! That's *really* important to me." And you may come to another and wonder, "Why would anyone care about that?" By checking out your reactions, you can redo the list to your own specifications, dropping some items, placing others at the very top of the list, and noting still others lower down. Now you're armed with a checklist to use in deciding among possible healers.

Still, many people today would find this advice a waste of time, because who has a choice any more over which healer to go to, especially in the case of regular physicians? In these days of managed care and limited choices, who gets to pick and choose?

Do I Have a Choice?

I want to offer my understanding and sympathy to the individuals for whom selecting a healer isn't a viable option. People on Medicaid or with no insurance may indeed have almost no choice of healers. Others may have a choice of only one insurance plan through their employer, which may be extremely restrictive in its allowable range of physicians.

For many, if not most, other people, more choice may actually be available than they first thought. I'll use my own practice as an example. I work in a group practice with about a dozen family physicians and three physician's assistants. We're signed up with all the managed care plans in our community, so any patient on any of those plans has an option to select us. In addition, most plans offer at least half a dozen choices of practices similar to ours. Once inside our practice, patients can also switch primary physicians. Someone who doesn't get along well with me can ask to be changed to any one of my eleven partners. Across the country, my clinic's situation is far from unique.

In managed care, you're often restricted in your choice of specialists. If you need to see a neurosurgeon or have special retinal surgery for an eye problem, there may be only one physician in your community available to you, and your insurance could refuse to cover costs if you leave town to seek care in another city. If you do have a choice of specialists and can pick one who has a number of the attributes on our list, all the better. Ideally, your primary physician can go to bat for you and help you find a specialist with the attributes that you most favor. Don't let this limit which applies to specialists discourage you from exercising other health options you actually do have.

Now I'm going to stick my neck out (given my bias as a family physician) and suggest that your choice of a primary physician or healer—with whom you will form an ongoing relationship and whom you will see first for the vast majority of health care issues—is, over the long haul, going to have a much greater impact on your inner pharmacy than is a specialist you'll use only for a single surgery or procedure. Though many people today consider managed care the enemy, smart insurance plans are actually on your side when it comes to choosing the best primary physician for your personal needs.

These insurance plans run more smoothly and ultimately spend a lot less money when you and your primary physician trust each other and have the best working relationship. Often managed care plans will allow free get-acquainted visits with your proposed new physician to allow you to check things out and be sure you want to go to that office. By contrast, in the pre-managed-care days, that visit would come out of your own pocket. In addition, managed care plans are beginning to provide patients with much more information about the various physicians in their plans.

Let's say you've selected a healer who seems right for you. What can you do to best prepare yourself for the encounter with her? Even if you felt unable to exercise much free choice in selecting your healer, don't despair just yet—it's possible that if you prepare well for each visit, that healer will turn out to be a better "fit" than you thought at first.

Planning Your Visit

One key element of the meaning model, as we've repeatedly stressed, is mastery or control. Some people imagine that as soon as they decide to go to a healer, control goes out the window; since by seeking help, you're giving up control. I feel that either-or reasoning is quite mistaken. You should be able to seek help for your problems and still develop an enhanced sense of mastery. You ought to feel more in control precisely because you took the initiative to seek help. As I've mentioned, the wrong sort of healer might end up robbing you of that sense of control. If you use the checklist of questions, you greatly diminish the odds of this happening.

When planning each visit with your chosen healer, your agenda should include the following parts. We'll assume for now that you are seeing a conventional physician, but the plan could easily be modified if you are consulting an alternative practitioner.

- What do I need to tell the physician about what has happened since my last visit?
- What questions about my health or about my treatment do I need to have answered?
- What do I hope to have happen as a result of the visit? What can I do to make sure that these things occur?
- What needs to happen on this visit to ensure that the long-term relationship with the physician is strengthened and directed in the right way?

This list doesn't imply a struggle for power with the physician, or a need for you to take total control over the relationship. If the physician interprets it that way, despite your best efforts, you may need to go back to the instructions for how to choose a healer. The goal is one of sharing control rather than taking over control. The physician or healer, after all, knows a lot about sickness and health and a lot about how to practice her craft. It definitely wouldn't be to your advantage to try to seize control in a way that undermines what the healer can do to help you.

To prepare for the visit, you may want to write your questions down and to bring the list with you. Physicians who become upset when patients bring in lists of questions, or who label all patients with lists as neurotics or hypochondriacs, are probably not the sort you want to be working with. Once at the visit itself, you still need to take a certain degree of control to make sure that your part of the agenda is taken care of.

Remember, you'll need to ask questions. You'll need to speak up right away if you don't understand or disagree with something. You'll need to fight against complacency and intimidation when something is unclear or the visit is going in a direction you don't like.

As I mentioned earlier, there may simply not be time to cover everything on your list, plus everything the physician feels is necessary. Schedule a follow-up visit to be sure all your issues are addressed. Work determinedly with the physician to make sure that future visits are long enough to deal with what is necessary. Even if this means higher costs for you in the short run, it will ultimately produce the best health results.

When the visit is over, your physician is going to make some notes about it for the medical chart, while it's fresh in her mind. You should do the same. Start jotting down ideas of what needs to happen on the next visit while you're still clear about the one you just had. What worked best? What didn't work so well? How can you make things function more smoothly on the next visit?

One way to be sure you're fully prepared is to rehearse your visit with the healer.

The Value of Rehearsal

This process of rehearsing for a visit to the doctor can be important for two reasons. First, as we've seen, it's basically mastery advice, which will enhance your healing sense of control. Second, as we talked about in chapter 13, it's an opportunity for you to do story work. By practicing your story before the visit, you may receive benefits which extend beyond simply being better prepared.

As a family physician, I periodically see patients who announce at the start of the appointment that they are already cured and don't need my help. The reason turns out to be that in the process of rehearsal, the patient has for the first time really analyzed his story, which has led him to his own insights about the cause and the cure of his condition. Here's a sample dialogue from such a visit between a doctor and a patient:

Doctor: I see that you wanted to talk to me about your diarrhea.

Patient: Yes, that's why I made the appointment, but now I'm embarrassed to be here taking up your time.

D: Why? Isn't the diarrhea a problem?

P: Yes, but you see, while I was driving over here today I thought I'd better get ready for your visit by going over in my head all the questions you were likely to ask me. And so I started telling myself all the things I knew about why my diarrhea was worse lately, when for years the diet changes you prescribed seemed to be working just great.

And then I realized that just about the time the diarrhea started to get worse, a new employee was transferred into my department. I've had a lot of conflicts with him, but I didn't want to make waves, so I haven't said anything. And that reminded me about a time six years ago when I had a flare-up of the diarrhea, and it came when I was under stress at work. Back then, the diarrhea finally got better when I got up the courage to talk to my supervisor. It was really hard for me to do that; but in the end it helped a lot. So now I think I know just exactly what I need to do to deal with this new episode of my same old problem.

D: Well, that's terrific. I'm delighted that I can't do anything for you!

In this particular case, the patient's story not only provided a solid explanation for the problem, but also pointed to a solution. We could predict that it's highly likely that the patient's diarrhea will start to get better even before he speaks to his supervisor, as this sort of positive change in meaning is often just what it takes to turn on the inner pharmacy full blast.

Of course, it's too much to expect all symptoms to disappear simply because we rehearse for the visit with the healer, but it never hurts to jump-start the placebo response and the inner pharmacy by taking this opportunity to go over your story in advance.

The Importance of Relationships

In current medical journals, you can find articles employing such terms as "sustained partnership" and "participatory decision-making model." These articles are appearing because the newest scientific evidence strongly suggests that patients' health improves the most within a certain form of relationship.

Exactly what form of relationship is this? Dr. Nancy Leopold and colleagues at the Agency for Health Care Policy and Research defined the term *sustained partnership* with the following list of characteristics, many of which you'll recognize from our previous discussions:

- The physician is interested in the whole person, and how all health-related problems relate to each other and to the patient's life.

- The physician knows the patient over time, not just the medical history, but the person's family life, work experiences, and basic values and preferences.

- The physician displays ongoing caring, sensitivity, and empathy in the relationship.

- The patient has found the physician to be credible and reliable over time and therefore has a substantial level of trust that the physician will act in the patient's best interests.

- The physician adapts the medical goals of care to the patient's unique needs, based on the patient's life goals and values as well as his social and cultural situation.

- The patient is encouraged to participate fully in health decision-making, and key medical decisions are shared between physician and patient.

Leopold and her colleagues selected this list because they found evidence in scientific studies that patients in those sorts of relationships had measurable improvements in their health as a result. That is, the relationship is a can't-lose proposition.

When we discussed modern brain science in chapter 9, we saw that important human relationships are assuming a role in today's theories of brain function and brain chemistry. The human brain, as I've said, is a superb ignoring machine. One way it marks a message to which we should pay attention is by sending it to us attached to an important human relationship. The more we can form the right sort of supportive human relationship with a healer over time, the more likely it is that he'll be able to phone in prescriptions to our inner pharmacy.

By identifying acquiescence as the one personality variable that seems to predict the positive placebo responder, Seymour Fisher and Roger Greenberg are indirectly emphasizing the importance of the sustained partnership as the best way to turn on the inner pharmacy. They quote, for example, one study of depressed patients, some of whom were receiving an antidepressant medication and some a placebo. All were also seeing a therapist. Videotapes were made of a visit with the therapist. Observers were asked to rate the tapes according to how good a therapeutic alliance existed between the therapist and that particular patient. The strength of the alliance proved to be an excellent predictor of getting better, and that was true both for patients getting the placebo, and those getting the "active" drug.

These sorts of findings led Fisher and Greenberg to state that what seemed to be especially important about the acquiescent patient was not meekness or impressionability, but a willingness to form good social relationships and to use others as resources in problem-solving. The acquiescent patient, in other words, seems to be the sort of person who would be a good candidate for forming a sustained partnership with a healer.

Physicians and healers ought to try to promote the sustained-partnership form of relationship. Since it's a two-way street, that also means that you have to assume some of the responsibility. After all, for the bond to be sustained and for it to be a partnership, you too have to work at it. Taking a reasonable degree of control over the relationship with the physician or healer is a part of the overall task of taking reasonable control over your own health.

Granted, this book is about the placebo response and the inner pharmacy, not health policy and health economics. But before I leave the subject of the ideal relationship between the patient and the healer, I want to say a few words about the broader implications of the model of care we have been discussing in this chapter.

Good News for a Better Health Care System

If we gathered a group of thoughtful people and talked for a while about what sort of health care system this country needs, I suspect they would eventually arrive at a list like this:

- Scientific medicine
- Humane medicine

- Personalized medicine
- Ethical medicine
- Affordable medicine

One reason so many people feel deeply frustrated with our present health care system is that these desirable features seem to be on a mutual collision course. For instance, all too often, modern scientific medicine seems increasingly inhumane and impersonal. As medicine becomes more technologically advanced, it also becomes unaffordable. So the mechanisms we have used to keep down costs, managed care for example, seem today to be producing inhumane, depersonalized, and occasionally unethical medicine. Is there any way out of this tangle?

The hard truth is that to some extent trade-offs are inevitable. With advances in science and technology, health care does get more expensive. As the average age of the population increases, people require more medical care. It's likely that in the future we'll either have to pay more or get less. Nor is it clear that the increased use of alternative medicine will do much to bring down costs, since most Americans use alternative medicine in addition to, rather than in place of, conventional care.

Before you get too discouraged, let's imagine that we were about to start afresh in designing our health care system, in such a way that the sustained partnership was at the very center. What would this mean?

First, it would be good scientific medicine, because as we saw, there is evidence that more people get better faster when they have this sort of medical care. When the basic relationship itself, and the remedies used by the primary physician, failed to make you better, then your partner would of course seek to obtain for you the best scientific options, including consultations with specialists and more extensive testing.

Second, most people would see this philosophy of medicine as being humane and personalized. The healer providing your care would be someone you know and trust who is dedicated to helping you over the long haul. Instead of employers' changing managed care contracts every year and demanding that you find a new primary care physician each time, this system would place the highest priority on maintaining long-term relationships.

Third, this new system would meet the modern standards for ethical care. If you go back and look at the elements of sustained partnership, you'll see that it demands that patients be active participants in choosing what care they want and be fully informed about their options. In this relationship, as we've discussed, you would have rights that allow you to choose on your own; and you would also have someone to lean on when you want help or advice.

Fourth, there's good reason to think that this system would be somewhat more affordable than our present state of affairs. The physicians who would be central to this plan, primary care physicians, tend to charge lower fees than the specialists who dominate the medical field today. It's generally less expensive to buy more time to communicate with your primary physician than to buy more lab tests and X rays, days in the hospital, surgical procedures, or consultations with specialists. Evidence also suggests that when the doctor who sees you for a problem is familiar with your medical history, the diagnosis and treatment can be much more carefully targeted toward what you need and, in addition, will cost less than if a stranger saw you. When your primary care physician does refer you for special tests or consultations, they will be used more selectively and logically than they are today.

If we're determined to undertake a serious reform of our health care system but want to guarantee the essential quality of care, here's a way to do it: Start with the idea of the sustained partnership as the hub of the wheel and work from there. In short, if we let the placebo response and the inner pharmacy do more of the work of healing, the bill from the outer pharmacy will be considerably less costly.

Epilogue: The Mystery of Healing

A Brief Review

Let's see what we've learned so far.

- In the past half-century, medical science has amassed substantial knowledge about the *placebo response.* It's a powerful and pervasive force in healing that is *not* restricted to the use of sugar pills or to deception.
- It's helpful to think of the placebo response in connection with the image of an *inner pharmacy*—as the science of the placebo response seems to be telling us that the body is capable of healing itself much of the time by releasing its own internal chemicals. Certain types of healing messages seem to be capable of turning on this inner pharmacy and enhancing its activity.
- The messages that most effectively stimulate the inner pharmacy change what the illness *means* to us. A positive change in meaning occurs when we feel that the illness has been explained; that we are surrounded by those who care for us; and that we can exercise mastery and control over what is bothering us.
- Humans attach meaning to events by *telling stories* about those events, and the inner pharmacy is highly responsive to the kinds of stories we construct about our health and illnesses. By telling a

story with a better ending, we can change meaning and hence stimulate the inner pharmacy.

- We are making progress in identifying the chemical pathways in the body by which the inner pharmacy might work. Future research with brain imaging might expand our understanding of the meaning-making centers of the brain and how they are linked to the endorphin, stress/relaxation, and psychoneuroimmune pathways.
- The placebo response and the inner pharmacy are not restricted to either conventional or alternative medicine. They form an intersection where different schools of healing meet. You can obtain the benefits of the inner pharmacy no matter which of the many types of treatment you employ.
- Once you understand the nature of the inner pharmacy and the methods by which you attach meaning to health and illness events, you'll be able to use the knowledge to bolster your health. You can do this in partnership with a healer and on your own. The last five chapters have shown you some specific techniques that will prove useful to healing the mind-body in either situation.

Our Enigmatic Bodies and Minds

This journey into medical science began with a mystery: the mystery of the sugar pill. Twentieth-century medical science thought it had successfully banished the mind from the healing process, and that, by breaking the body down into its tiniest components, it would soon cure all disease and extend healthy life. That strategy left scientists unable to account for a very basic fact: that people got better—in terms both of how they felt and how their bodies functioned—after taking pills which could not possibly have had any direct chemical or physiological effect on their condition. To try to explain this mystery, modern medical science had no other choice than to find some means to reintroduce the human mind into the equation of medicine and healing. Modern neuroscience insists that's how it should have been all along, that it is a grotesque misunderstanding of the human body to imagine we could somehow eliminate the mind from consideration when explaining human health and illness.

The need to explain this mystery led inevitably to new mysteries. The major enigma of the placebo response is its individual unpredictability. We have seen that on average about a third of people tested respond to a placebo stimulus. This apparent average masks marked variation. In some circumstances, there is almost no placebo response; and in other situations, especially those of heightened expectancy, the placebo response may rise to 70 to 80 percent. Efforts to identify a placebo-responder personality type, and predict with any sort of confidence exactly who will respond to placebos and under what circumstances, have generally failed. The exception was the personality trait of acquiescence, which among other things may predict who is best at forming solid interpersonal relationships with others.

This lack of predictability may appear extremely discouraging to anyone intent on promoting the placebo response as a tool in healing. After all, who wants to trust a protocol that works on average merely a third of the time? This "bad news" pertains only if we ignore another fact about healing: namely, that no treatment in medicine is 100 percent reliable or predictable. Antibiotics for pneumonia, chemotherapy for cancer, surgery for clogged arteries: All have a statistical failure rate and saddle practitioners with the inability to predict in advance for whom any given treatment will succeed or fail.

Knowing that the only difference between the placebo response and other forms of treatment is the size of the success rate, we can decide to employ it as a healing tool under the following conditions:

- We do so honestly.
- The risk of causing harm is extremely low.
- Using the placebo response does not preclude employing any other form of treatment.

- Using the placebo response adds very little to the cost of care (or even reduces the cost).

All these conditions apply most of the time when we use the placebo response in accordance with the meaning model. It seems fruitless to argue about whether we should attempt to use the response's healing potential. We would be foolish not to try. This is especially true when the placebo response, ignored or neglected, has the potential to turn into a *nocebo response*, which will actually make us worse.

Puzzles and Mysteries

We do not like mysteries and much prefer puzzles. A puzzle is something to which we do not know the answer, but to which the answer can be known, and for which we have a procedure that is more or less certain to lead us eventually to the answer. What we call "mystery novels" are actually puzzle novels: If at the end of the novel we still don't know whether or not the butler did it, we feel cheated.

Medicine has made great progress in our century by treating disease as a puzzle—and, granted, the puzzle approach is extremely effective within limits. I suggest it will be important in discovering what portions of the brain are involved in assigning meaning to events, and how those portions of the brain are connected to various biochemical pathways. Further research on the stories we tell about illness and how changing their endings may ultimately alter our state of health will also be productive. These are puzzles. They can be solved.

A true mystery, by contrast, cannot be solved. In the end, you have only to acknowledge and devise a way to live with it. If this sounds odd—and indeed seems almost antiscientific or anti-intellectual—it's because our modern culture has become so firmly committed to the myth of progress that we've completely neglected the ancient concept of mystery. We make progress, after all, by trying to change things and solve puzzles. We assume we cannot make progress by simply accepting things as they are.

Perhaps the classic presentation of the true meaning of mystery is the Biblical story of Job. It is important in a healing sense as well as a religious one because God's testing of Job entailed not only the loss of his children and all his possessions, but also his bodily health. Job's friends, and later Job himself, attempt to approach what has happened to him as a puzzle. The friends claim God never punishes those who are blameless, so Job must have done something to offend Him, possibly without knowing it at the time. If they could pinpoint the offense, they would understand why Job is being punished.

Job knows that such reasoning is nonsense. But when he speaks to God directly, he still seeks a solution to a puzzle, assuming he is entitled to one. God's reply to Job is a rebuke—not for having offended Him by sinning (for indeed Job is blameless of that); but rather for failing to understand Him as mystery.

The interpretations of the Job story which I find most compelling see God as saying to Job that, because he is a human being, he's not entitled to an answer to the puzzle because God is mystery. It's contradictory to say you worship God, and then demand an answer from Him as if He were a puzzle. Instead, true worship requires accepting God as fundamentally mysterious. What befalls mortals may also be mysterious, and the mystery, in some cases, may be that terrible things happen to blameless people.

Such statements as, "I will worship you, God, but only if you promise no evil will ever befall me as long as I do good," or, "I will worship you, God, but only if you guarantee me a complete explanation if anything evil that happens in the world seemingly as a result of your will" actually constitute a refusal to worship Him. At the end of Job's story, he is indeed healed, but only when he accepts mystery and gives up trying to solve puzzles.

I have spoken of meaning and mastery as keys to understanding the placebo response. Taken by themselves, these two concepts may suggest that all we have to do, in order to stimulate our inner pharmacies for healing, is to solve puzzles. I must now balance the account by adding mystery as a third important key to triggering the inner pharmacy. Sometimes the most healing thing to do will be to construct meaning and establish mastery; but other times, it will be to understand and accept mystery.

The "Quarter-in-the-Slot" Trap

Not only conventional medicine endeavors to dispense with mysteries and stick to puzzles. I have seen this same tendency in many books on alternative medicine, mind-body healing, and New Age thought. Much of this writing seems to possess what I referred to in the introduction as the "quarter-in-the-slot" mentality. If you follow this specific recipe or formula, you need only turn the knob to be healed, with the same degree of certitude that you'll get a gumball out of a gumball machine. If you aren't healed, it must be your own fault. Obviously you didn't follow the recipe or formula correctly. At this point, I want to make sure you don't fall into this mental trap. Indeed, if I'm not completely clear on this point, I'll be jeopardizing the entire ethical—and healing—basis on which this book was constructed.

Part of the unfortunate stigma attached to the word "placebo" is, as we know, that it began as a form of lying. For centuries, physicians gave patients dummy medicines of one sort or another—remember the dummy enema Montaigne described in 1580 and the bread pills of which Thomas Jefferson wrote in 1807—and either told the patients, or allowed them to think, they were getting an entirely different substance. I have tried in this book to rehabilitate the placebo response by associating it with truth and candor rather than lies. If you try to change the meaning of illness for yourself, or tell yourself a better story, you can do so knowing exactly what you're up to. The inner pharmacy, after all, is just as capable of responding to truthful messages as to lies, if not more so.

My truth-in-advertising pitch is this: No advice in this book should be taken as any sort of recipe or guarantee for successful healing. There are a number of puzzles about the placebo response that will be solved with further research. And there are puzzles about yourself and your response to illness that you can solve with careful inquiry. But, at its heart, the placebo response is destined always to remain at least partly a mystery. It will not work fully for us as a healing response unless we understand and accept this.

I am not saying that the placebo response is unpredictable simply as a way of getting myself off the hook if it doesn't work for you precisely as you would wish. I am saying that I want the experience of reading this book to be a healing sort of experience for you—just as I think that your experience of the ideal practitioner should involve being in the presence of "a healing sort of person." If I haven't managed to convey to you the importance of mystery, then I will have failed to portray true healing.

This leads to a central paradox: The more desperately you want and demand healing, the less likely you are to be healed. Healing in this regard is somewhat like love. If you are truly desperate for a person to love, and approach each encounter with another as a quest for the life partner of your dreams, you are almost sure to repel anyone who is even vaguely eligible and nip any love relationship in the bud. The people who successfully meet others and fall mutually in love in a satisfying way are usually the least desperate and the most confident in their ability to go on living by themselves if that is what fate has in store for them. It is this very confidence that draws eligible partners.

Still, there are times when everybody's confidence flags. What then?

Conquering Doubt with Hope

Caroline Myss wrote, "Our lives are made up of a series of mysteries that we are meant to explore but that are meant to remain unsolved." Nowhere is this more true than in healing, the placebo response, the mind-body connection, and in facing our own mortality. What are we supposed to do when we have been prescribed a treatment for some illness? Expectancy theory teaches us that the more we expect and believe the treatment will work, the greater the chance that we'll have the inner pharmacy on our side. We try to think positive thoughts, but then the doubting sets in.

There are two things we could tell ourselves when the doubts begin.

At first glance, they might seem almost identical, but I suggest that they are profoundly different. One is, "Doggone it, I have to get rid of these doubts! The treatment will never work if I don't get my mind working positively in sync with my body. So I have to banish these doubts or the inner pharmacy will never work." Viewing hope and expectancy in this fashion is to fall back into the quarter-in-the-slot trap, which tends to discourage, rather than promote healing.

The second reaction to doubt is that it's natural. "After all," you tell yourself, "I have no way of knowing whether in the end this treatment will or won't work. But I do know that hope increases the odds of its working in my favor. So let's see what I can do to summon hope. And let me try to do that without getting into any blaming, punishment, or bargaining games. After all, it's not just a question of whether or not I will be cured. It's a question of what sort of person I want to be, and of what sort of story I want to tell about my life. And I have to decide if, when push comes to shove, I want to be a hopeful person or a doubting person."

This second way of thinking is much more healing because it accepts and deals with mystery, then moves beyond the mystery into action. The action is all the more confident and hopeful precisely because it accepts the mystery of healing and makes no attempt to deny or evade it.

Take the case of Felix:

Felix

Felix is a fifty-year-old physician and teacher, as well as a personal friend of mine. Three years ago, he was diagnosed with cancer of the esophagus, a very odd and unexpected diagnosis for a person so young. He had surgery to correct the blockage, but at the time he was not given much hope for long-term remission.

My friend was married with young children, making the prognosis even more tragic. He responded to the cancer by defining it as a wake-up call forcing him to confront his mortality, which, up until now, he'd never really considered. Now he thought about it a lot, finally coming to terms with what it would mean to leave his family and his life activities. He was especially concerned with how to live each day to the fullest, knowing it might be one of his last. He ultimately concluded there was much pleasure in life he had previously denied himself, because he had always been too busy to live fully in the present.

After accepting impending death, Felix set about living as healthy a life as he could, making major changes in his diet and exercise regimen. He was at peace with his choices, since he didn't want to die and was willing to invest a lot of energy in trying to live longer. If an early death awaited him, he was at peace with the prospect. What he refused to do was expend his energy in fear.

Since then, two things have happened. First, Felix has become an inspiration to all his friends, describing his cancer as a "gift" which has allowed him truly to live for the first time. Second, he is now about two years beyond the most optimistic of the early predictions for his length of survival.

Felix seems to me to be a wonderful example of healing by accepting mystery. His very presence seems incredibly healing to others since he takes joy in his friendships and in the simple pleasures of living. For him, going down the street with his wife for a cappuccino is similar to a kid going to Disney World for the first time. Somehow he manages to convey this sense of joyfulness to everyone he meets and talks to. He conveys so much peace and healing to everyone else around him that I envision his inner pharmacy working overtime. I believe that if you gave Herbert Benson's relaxation response a body and dressed it in a suit of clothes, it would be Felix.

What I mean by the central paradox of the mystery of the placebo response is this: Felix has so much to live for that one could readily understand him becoming desperate and demanding a successful cure. He could easily start on a tour of the best hospitals and the best alternative healing centers, looking at each place for the guarantee that he's going to lick his cancer. But he has not done this. He seems to have gained healing precisely to the degree with which he faced and made peace with dying. Many desperate patients devote so much of their energy to keeping the very idea of death at a distance that they have little energy left over for real healing. Felix let go of his fears so thoroughly that all of his energy could be devoted to his health—and to loving his wife and children, which undoubtedly contributed to his own health as well. Felix, I suggest, helped to heal himself precisely to the extent that he accepted healing as mystery.

A Final Word

When we address the central paradox of the mystery of the placebo response, we always come back to the importance of meaning in our lives. We are forced to ask, in order to be as healthy as we can be, what sort of person do we want to become—that is, what do we want our lives to mean? If we're presently healthy, we're challenged to decide how to keep on being as healthy as we can while still engaging in all the other projects and activities that make our lives meaningful. That is, we must refuse to narrow our lives by making health our only goal. If we are suffering from an illness right now, it dares us, as Arthur Frank likes to say, to "rise to the occasion"—to see what it would be like to go on living a meaningful life with the illness, even if its total elimination may not be a realistic prospect. Carl Jung is said to have written, "Meaning makes a good deal of things bearable—perhaps everything." And in the words of poet, playwright, and president of the Czech Republic Václav Havel:

> ***"Hope is definitely not the same thing as optimism. It is not the conviction that something will turn out well, but the certainty that something makes sense, regardless of how it turns out. . . . It is also this hope, above all, which gives us the strength to live and continually try new things . . . "***

In presenting the ideas in this book, I have tried to be both realistic and optimistic. My experience as a family physician and as a medical educator is that the healer and the patient, together in partnership, can really make a difference. For me, the optimism is genuine.

At this point, it's easy to be optimistic. I've seen the processes we've discussed work, as have countless physicians and scientists, many of whose experience and research you've read about in these pages. These means of healing don't often produce results as dramatic as, say, the faith healings at Lourdes. No, the paralyzed may not throw down their crutches and walk away unaided. Nonetheless the processes are effective at the level where most good medicine functions: People suffer less from the symptoms of their illness, discover they can do more despite their illness, and realize that, even with illness, their lives are meaningful.

When all this happens, I know that I am in the presence of healing. Just *how and why* it happens may remain a mystery. *That* it happens is as certain as anything can be in the practice of medicine.

Bibliographic Essay

This essay begins by listing general references on the placebo response. It then proceeds to indicate, chapter by chapter, the sources of information and quotations. Each citation begins with an italicized phrase, which is the passage from the text at the place where the citation is mentioned or is relevant.

General: Books and Articles About the Placebo Response

Books

A number of books, which vary widely in content and approach, have appeared about the placebo response since the 1970s.

A book which is not devoted solely to the placebo response, strictly speaking, but which deserves mention as a frequently quoted classic, is Jerome D. Frank, *Persuasion and Healing* (revised edition, Baltimore: Johns Hopkins University Press, 1973). Frank devotes one chapter to the placebo response. His main concern is to show what the various schools of psychotherapy have in common, and to argue that these shared elements are much more responsible for the success of psychotherapy than any individual technique prized by one school or another. The placebo response, as we define it in this book, is one of those common elements. Many of the healing strategies we discuss in chapters 12 through 16 are at least hinted at, if not specifically mentioned, by Frank.

Jefferson M. Fish, *Placebo Therapy* (San Francisco: Jossey-Bass,

1973), also focuses on the placebo response in psychotherapy. Fish is one of the first to offer an expansive definition of "placebo effect" to cover almost every aspect of human interaction within the healing environment. He emphasizes (in a way similar to Jerome Frank) how psychotherapy can heal in part by harnessing the faith of the patient and by employing powerful rituals of healing.

Michael Jospe, *The Placebo Effect in Healing* (Lexington, MA: Lexington Books/D.C. Heath, 1978), also focuses on the placebo response as a psychological phenomenon and draws mainly on work by psychologists. It does contain a good review of what was known about the placebo effect at the time.

My own *Placebos and the Philosophy of Medicine: Clinical, Conceptual, and Ethical Issues* (Chicago: University of Chicago Press, 1980), says more about theories of the mind-body relationship than anyone besides a philosopher would like to know. It does, however, introduce some of the key ideas in this book— the importance of symbols for understanding the impact of the placebo on the mind; why one should define *placebo response* independently of *placebo*; and the meaning model.

Placebo: Theory, Research, and Mechanisms, edited by Leonard White, Bernard Tursky, and Gary E. Schwartz (New York: Guilford Press, 1985), remains the meatiest technical compendium of data and analysis about the placebo effect, featuring twenty-five chapters and 447 pages. It takes an interdisciplinary approach, including work by physicians, philosophers, psychologists, anthropologists, pharmacologists, and others. The last chapter is the editors' comprehensive model of how these approaches must be consolidated in order to truly understand the placebo response. While much important research has been done since this book was published, it is still a valuable reference.

Howard M. Spiro, *Doctors, Patients, and Placebos* (New Haven: Yale University Press, 1986), is written by a physician and consequently focuses on the placebo response in clinical practice as well as in research. I find this volume somewhat inconsistent. In the earlier chapters Dr. Spiro tends to take a skeptical view of many of the claims made for the placebo effect. He insists upon a distinction that I find fallacious, arguing that the placebo is capable of changing subjective feelings of patients, but not of changing any objective measures of bodily function. (My chapter 9 explains to some extent why modern neuroscience would reject any subjective/objective distinction of this sort.) His later chapters, by contrast, are a very sensitive presentation of the placebo response as an aid to the humane and compassionate physician-patient relationship. His key bit of concluding imagery is to contrast the eye and the ear. Modern medicine has enshrined the eye, hoping to learn the truth by gazing at the body either directly or through technology like X rays. But, Spiro says, the placebo needs the ear. Human listening needs to be restored as a critical part of medicine. Spiro revised and expanded his discussion in a later volume, *The Power of Hope: A Doctor's Perspective* (New Haven, CT: Yale University Press, 1998).

Non-Specific Aspects of Treatment, edited by Michael Shepherd and Norman Sartorius (Lewiston, NY: Hans Huber Publishers, 1989), a publication of the World Health Organization, is essentially a collection of five essays, representing the disciplines of philosophy of science, experimental psychology, clinical pharmacology, psychotherapy, and clinical psychiatry. Thus Shepherd and Sartorius continue the strategy begun by White, Tursky, and Schwartz of studying the placebo response from an interdisciplinary point of view.

This same strategy is continued in *The Placebo Effect: An Interdisciplinary Exploration,* edited by Anne Harrington (Cambridge, MA: Harvard University Press, 1997). The volume grew out of a conference held in 1994 at Harvard, and includes both formal papers by participants and also some of the give-and-take discussion in between. The papers in this book are uniformly of very high quality and extremely thought-provoking.

Arthur K. Shapiro and Elaine Shapiro, *The Powerful Placebo: From Ancient Priest to Modern Physician* (Baltimore: Johns Hopkins University Press, 1997), summarizes the life's work of one of the most prolific modern writers on the placebo effect, psychiatrist Arthur Shapiro. Sadly, Dr. Shapiro died before the book was completed, and the volume seems to be more a collection of his previous articles on the placebo effect than a comprehensive reanalysis. Dr. Shapiro, like Dr. Spiro, apparently felt toward the end of his life that more claims were being made for the placebo effect than could be scientifically validated.

While this volume is not easily available, I have benefited from reading the doctoral thesis *Placebos and Placebo Effects in Clinical Trials,* by Ton de Craen (Department of Clinical Epidemiology and Biostatistics, University of Amsterdam, 1998). Many of the individual chapters have been published in medical journals and will be cited.

One recent book, *The Placebo Response: Biology and Belief in Clinical Practice,* a collection of essays edited by D. Peters (London: Churchill Livingstone, 1999), became available too late for me to review for this volume.

Technical Review Articles

During this same time period, there have been a great number of review articles about the placebo response in medical journals and other technical publications. What follows is a selected rather than complete list.

One of the very first such articles, and one we shall refer back to often below, is Henry K. Beecher, "The Powerful Placebo," *Journal of the American Medical Association* 159:1602–1606, 1955.

Other valuable articles include Stewart Wolf, "The Pharmacology of Placebos," *Pharmacological Review* 2:689–704, 1959; Arthur K. Shapiro, "The Placebo Response," in *Modern Perspectives in World Psychiatry,* edited by J.G. Howells (Edinburgh: Oliver and Boyd, 1968), pp. 596–619; Henry R. Bourne, "The Placebo—A Poorly Understood and Neglected Therapeutic Agent," *Rational Drug Therapy* 5(11):1–6, 1971; Herbert Benson and Mark D. Epstein, "The Placebo Effect: A Neglected Asset in the Care of Patients," *Journal of the American Medical Association* 232:1225–1227, 1975; Alfred O. Berg, "Placebos: A Brief Review for Family Physicians," *Journal of Family Practice* 5:97–100, 1977; Henry R. Bourne, "Rational Use of Placebo," in *Clinical Pharmacology: Basic Principles in Therapeutics* (second edition), edited by Kenneth L. Melmon and Howard F. Morrelli (New York: Macmillan, 1978); Arthur K. Shapiro and Louis A. Morris, "The Placebo Effect in Medical and

Psychological Therapies," in *Handbook of Psychotherapy and Behavior Change: An Empirical Analysis* (second edition), edited by S.L. Garfield and A.E. Bergin (New York: Wiley, 1978), pp. 369–419; Vernon Min Sen Oh, "Magic or Medicine? Clinical Pharmacological Basis of Placebo Medication," *Annals of the Academy of Medicine (Singapore)* 20:31–37, 1991; and Judith A. Turner, Richard A. Deyo, John D. Loeser, Michael Von Korff, and Wilbert E. Fordyce, "The Importance of Placebo Effects in Pain Treatment and Research," *Journal of the American Medical Association* 271:1609–1614, 1994.

In 1994, *The Lancet* published a series of articles on the placebo response in its Volume 344. These included D. Mark Chaput de Saintonge and Andrew Herxheimer, "Harnessing Placebo Effects in Health Care," pp. 995–998; K. B. Thomas, "The Placebo in General Practice," pp. 1066–1067; Alan A. Johnson, "Surgery as a Placebo," pp. 1140–1142; Joan-Ramon Laporte, "Placebo Effects in Psychiatry," pp. 1206–1209; and Jos Kleijnen, Anton J.M. de Craen, Jannes van Everdingen, and Leendert Krol, "Placebo Effect in Double-Blind Clinical Trials: A Review of Interactions with Medications," pp. 1347–1349.

An excellent comprehensive review, which I shall refer to numerous times, is by Seymour Fisher and Roger P. Greenberg, "The Curse of the Placebo: Fanciful Pursuit of a Pure Biological Therapy," in the book edited by these two authors, *From Placebo to Panacea: Putting Psychiatric Drugs to the Test* (New York: Wiley, 1997). This book takes the stance that most drugs commonly used today in psychiatry cannot be shown, upon careful investigation, to be any better than placebos. Regardless of what one thinks of this controversial thesis, their review of what is known about the placebo response is impressive.

Articles in Popular Magazines

Several articles on the placebo effect have appeared at intervals in *Scientific American;* see for instance Louis Lasagna, "Placebos," *Scientific American* 193 (July, 1956):68–71; and Walter A. Brown, "The Placebo Effect," *Scientific American,* Volume 278, Number 1, January 1998, pp. 90–95. Norman Cousins contributed "The Mysterious Placebo: How

Mind Helps Medicine Work," to the *Saturday Review*, October 1, 1977, pp. 9–16. *Psychology Today* has printed good reviews of the placebo response; see for example Frederick J. Evans, "The Power of the Sugar Pill," *Psychology Today* 7 (April 1974):55–59. An excellent recent assessment of current placebo research is Sandra Blakeslee, "Placebos Prove So Powerful Even Experts Are Surprised," *New York Times*, Science section, pp. 1–4, October 13, 1998.

Introduction: The Power of the Mind

xiv *Danielle has just had surgery to remove her gall bladder:* While this example may seem fanciful, one scientific study looked at healing after surgery as a function of the view out the patient's window: Roger S. Ulrich, "View Through a Window May Influence Recovery From Surgery," *Science* 224:420–421, 1984.

Chapter One: What Is the Placebo Response?

1 *"One of the most successful physicians":* The quotation is from *The Writings of Thomas Jefferson,* edited by P. L. Ford (New York: Putnam, 1898), Vol. IX, p. 78–85.

2 *Mr. Wright, Krebiozen, and the Newspaper Headlines:* The story of Mr. Wright appears in Bruno Klopfer, "Psychological Variables in Human Cancer," *Journal of Projective Techniques* 21:331–340, 1957.

3 *Ruth's Rose Perfume:* This case was published by Karen Olness and Robert Ader, "Conditioning as an Adjunct in the Pharmacotherapy of Lupus Erythematosus," *Journal of Developmental and Behavioral Pediatrics* 13:124–125, 1992.

4 *The Importance of Listening:* Martin J. Bass, Carol Buck, Linda Turner, et al., "The Physician's Actions and the Outcome of Illness in Family Practice," *Journal of Family Practice* 23:43–47, 1986.

4 *Bass and colleagues also identified a large group:* The Headache Study Group of the University of Western Ontario, "Predictors of Outcome in Headache Patients Presenting to Family Physicians—A One Year Prospective Study," *Headache Journal* 26:285–294, 1986.

5 *Consider that Barbara Starfield of Johns Hopkins University:* Barbara Starfield, Christine Wray, Kelliann Hess, et al., "The Influence of Patient-Practitioner Agreement on Outcome of Care," *American Journal of Public Health* 71:127–132, 1981.

5 *A Woman Who Died of Abbreviation:* Dr. Bernard Lown recounted this episode in his introduction to Norman Cousins's book, *The Healing Heart* (New York, Norton, 1983). In turn, Howard Spiro cited the anecdote in his *Doctors, Patients, and Placebos* (New Haven: Yale University Press, 1986), p. 247.

9 *So I can now expand my definition of* placebo response: In *Placebos and the Philosophy of Medicine: Clinical, Conceptual, and Ethical Issues* (Chicago: University of Chicago Press, 1980), I first introduced the importance of symbol-using as it relates to the concept of the placebo response, but the actual formation of a definition based on this idea came with my "Placebo Effect: An Examination of Grünbaum's Definition," in *Placebo: Theory, Research, and Mechanisms,* edited by Leonard White, Bernard Tursky, and Gary E. Schwartz (New York: Guilford Press, 1985), pp. 37–58.

10 *Some experts have suggested that one cannot define it in any logically coherent way:* Peter C. Gøtzsche, "Is There Logic in the Placebo?" *The Lancet* 344:925–926, 1994; Irving Kirsch, "Unsuccessful Redefinitions of the Term *Placebo,*" *American Psychologist* 41:844–845, 1986. A classic philosophical study of the definition of *placebo* is by Adolf Grünbaum, "Explication and Implications of the Placebo Concept," in *Placebo: Theory, Research, and Mechanisms,* edited by Leonard White, Bernard Tursky, and Gary E. Schwartz (New York: Guilford Press, 1985), pp. 9–36. Grünbaum's main contribution to the discussion was to point out how the definition of *placebo* or *placebo effect* is always tied to a specific medical theory, so that if our theory of "what works" changes, we will change also our view of what counts as a placebo. My own reactions to this approach are contained in "Placebo Effect: An Examination of Grünbaum's Definition," in the same volume, pp. 37–58. See also Joseph W. Critelli and Karl F. Neumann, "The Placebo: Conceptual Analysis of a Concept in Transition," *American Psychologist* 39:32–39, 1984.

12 *The placebo response is not nonspecific:* I owe this point to the writings of Irving Kirsch. See for example his "Specifying Nonspecifics: Psychological Mechanisms of Placebo Effects," in *The Placebo Effect: An Interdisciplinary Exploration,* edited by Anne Harrington (Cambridge, MA: Harvard University Press, 1997), pp. 166–186.

13 *You'll notice that so far, we have been defining placebo response*: I tried to justify this "backward" approach (defining placebo response first and placebo afterward) at some length in *Placebos and the Philosophy of Medicine: Clinical, Conceptual, and Ethical Issues* (Chicago: University of Chicago Press, 1980), pp. 25–44.

14 *By defining our terms in such a way that:* I first began to develop this connection between the approach to the definition and the ethics of using the placebo response in medical practice in "Commentary: On Placebos," *Hastings Center Report* 5(2):17–18, 1975. The classic paper, proposing that it is the physician and the overall healing context, and not the dummy pill, which is responsible for the placebo response, is W.R. Houston, "Doctor Himself as a Therapeutic Agent," *Annals of Internal Medicine* 11:1416–1425, 1938. See also Thomas Findley, "The Placebo and the Physician," *Medical Clinics of North America,* 37:1821–1826, 1953; and H. Keith Fischer and Barney M. Dlin, "The Dynamics of Placebo Therapy: A Clinical Study," *American Journal of the Medical Sciences* 232:504–512, 1956.

The Placebo Response: A Historical Perspective

16 *"Since almost all medications until recently":* Arthur K. Shapiro, "The Placebo Response," in *Modern Perspectives in World Psychiatry,* edited by J.G. Howells (Edinburgh: Oliver and Boyd, 1968), p. 597.

16 *The Rich Merchant's Magic Enema:* Michel de Montaigne, *Works* (Boston, Houghton Mifflin, 1880), Vol. I, p. 155.

17 *For us to learn as much as we can from that history:* There are a number of articles on the history of placebos and the placebo effect. The vast majority are *not* written by trained historians, and are really histories of therapies now considered to be ineffective. The articles provide a long list of therapies used in past times, which to us today sound silly, and conclude that since these silly treatments could not possibly have been effective chemically, their results (if any) must have been totally due to the placebo effect. These papers tell us nothing whatever about what physicians of that historical period actually thought about the relationship of mind and body in healing. Unfortunately, most of the "historical" writings of Arthur K. Shapiro (except for his work on the definition of *placebo* which I will soon address) fall into this category. A fairly typical article of this type is Donald W. Brodeur, "A Short History of Placebos," *Journal of the American Pharmaceutical Association* 5:642–643, 1965.

18 *The healing power of hope, faith, and the imagination . . . and the inherent healing power of the body itself.* Two classic historical works address these two sorts of explanations. On the power of the imagination, see Pedro Lain Entralgo, *The Therapy of the Word in Classical Antiquity,* edited and translated by L.J. Rather and John M. Sharp (New Haven: Yale University Press, 1970). On the healing power of nature, see Max Neuberger, *The Doctrine of the Healing Power of Nature Throughout the Course of Time,* translated by Linn J. Boyd, published in New York in 1932 (no publisher's imprint in the volume I examined).

18 *Again, a high value must be set upon truthfulness:* Plato, *The Republic,* (III.388) translated by F. M. Cornford (New York, Oxford University Press, 1945), p. 78.

19 *The free physician—the one who does not attend to slaves:* Plato, *Laws,* IV.720d-e.

19 *Because of the holism of humoral theory:* On the "fit" between the placebo concept and humoral medicine, see C.E. McMahon, "The Placebo Effect in Renaissance Medicine," *Journal of the American Society of Psychosomatic Dentistry and Medicine,* 22(1):3–9, 1975.

20 *[H]ope . . . buoys up a mind enfeebled:* Jerome Gaub, "Beneficial Corporeal Effects of Hope in Connection with Various Ailments," in L.J. Rather, *Mind and Body in Eighteenth Century Medicine: A Study Based on Jerome Gaub's De Regimine Mentis* (Berkeley, CA: University of California Press, 1965), p. 174.

20 *There is no virtue in such charms or cures:* Robert Burton, *The*

Anatomy of Melancholy (New York: Empire State Book Company, 1924), p. 168.

21 *The word "placebo" itself means:* The classic study of the evolution of the definition of *placebo* is Arthur K. Shapiro, "Semantics of the Placebo," *Psychiatric Quarterly,* 42:653–695, 1968. Louis Lasagna, in a review of Brody, *Placebos and the Philosophy of Medicine,* published in the *Bulletin of the History of Medicine,* Vol. 54, Winter 1980, pp. 613–615, suggests a solution to one historical puzzle: why the word *placebo* should appear at the start of the Latin version of Psalm 116. The correct rendition of the beginning of that Psalm is "I shall walk before the Lord . . ." Lasagna points out that the Hebrew version is indeed "et-ha-lech," which means "I shall walk." He suggests that the Hebrew was then mistranslated into the Septuagent Greek as "euaresteso," which was then "correctly" translated into the Vulgate Latin as "placebo," "I shall please."

21 *Dr. Franklin and Mr. Mesmer:* An excellent work on the history of blinded trials and placebo controls, which I have relied upon extensively, is Ted J. Kaptchuk, "Intentional Ignorance: A History of Blind Assessment and Placebo Controls in Medicine," *Bulletin of the History of Medicine* 72:389–433, 1998. The original report of Franklin's group is Benjamin Franklin et al., *Report of Dr. Benjamin Franklin, and Other Commissioners, Charged by the King of France, with the Examination of Animal Magnetism, as Now Practiced in Paris,* translated by William Godwin (London: J. Johnson, 1785).

22 *The Tractor Test:* John Haygarth, *Of the Imagination, as a Cause and as a Cure of Disorders of the Body; Exemplified by Fictitious Tractors and Epidemical Convulsions* (Bath: R. Cruttwell, 1801).

22 *The principal influence or relation of [drugs] to the cure:* Elmer Lee, "How Far Does a Scientific Therapy Depend Upon the Materia Medica in the Cure of Disease," *Journal of the American Medical Association,* Volume 31, October 8, 1898, p. 827 (quoted in: Charles E. Rosenberg, "The Therapeutic Revolution: Medicine, Meaning, and Social Change in Nineteenth Century America," in *The Therapeutic Revolution,* edited by Morris J. Vogel and Charles E. Rosenberg (Philadelphia: University of Pennsylvania Press, 1979), p. 19.

23 *Dr. Flint's Placeboic Remedy:* The report of this experiment is Austin Flint, "A Contribution Toward the Natural History of Articular Rheumatism," *American Journal of the Medical Sciences* 46(N.S.):2–36, 1863.

24 *As evidence accumulated through the nineteenth century:* Perhaps the most comprehensive work on this subject at the time was Daniel Hack Tuke, *Illustrations of the Influence of the Mind upon the Body in Health and Disease* (Philadelphia: Lea, 1873), especially pp. 367–371. Tuke, a pioneer student of psychiatry in England, was perhaps the inventor of what in later times became known as psychosomatic medicine. For his factual material, Tuke relied heavily on some case reports recorded by John Forbes. See for example "Notes of Some Experiments, Illustrating the Influence of the Vis Medicatrix, and of the Imagination, in the Cure of Diseases, by a Naval Surgeon, In a Letter to John Forbes, M.D., F.R.S.," *British and Foreign Medical Review* 23:265–269, 1847.

24 *Some time ago I gave to a patient:* Horatio C. Wood, "General Therapeutic Considerations," in *A System of Practical Therapeutics,* edited by Hobart A. Hare (Philadelphia: Lea, 1891), p. 42.

24 *Charles Rosenberg, a prominent medical historian, writes:* Charles E. Rosenberg, "The Therapeutic Revolution: Medicine, Meaning, and Social Change in Nineteenth Century America," in *The Therapeutic Revolution,* edited by Morris J. Vogel and Charles E. Rosenberg (Philadelphia: University of Pennsylvania Press, 1979), p. 16.

25 *Now I was brought up, as I suppose every physician is:* Richard C. Cabot, "The Use of Truth and Falsehood in Medicine: An Experimental Study," *American Medicine* 5:344–349, 1903.

25 *[At a recent meeting of the General Practice Section]:* "The Bottle of Medicine" (editorial), *British Medical Journal,* Volume 1, 1952, p. 149.

26 *Some branches of medical science have already attained:* "Medical Society of London," *The Lancet,* vol. 1 for 1855, p. 292.

26 *I knew a surgeon years ago who thought nothing:* Norman Shure, "The Placebo Effect in Allergy," *Annals of Allergy* 23:368–376, 1965.

27 *When a patient is suspected, then, to have no "real" bodily disease:* A useful modern study of the actual use of placebos in American teaching hospitals is James S. Goodwin, Jean M. Goodwin, and Albert V. Vogel, "Knowledge and Use of Placebos by House Officers and Nurses," *Annals of Internal Medicine* 91:106–110, 1979. See also Richard J. Goldberg, Hoyle Leigh, and Donald Quinlan, "The Current Status of Placebo in Hospital Practice," *General Hospital Psychiatry* 1:196–201, 1979; and Gerald Gray and Patrick Flynn, "A Survey of Placebo Use in a General Hospital," *General Hospital Psychiatry* 3:199–203, 1981.

28 *Ted Kaptchuk, who has surveyed this history carefully:* These arguments are to be found in Ted J. Kaptchuk, "Powerful Placebo: The Dark Side of the Randomized Controlled Trial," *The Lancet* 351:1722–1725, 1998.

29 *"The powerful placebo," as his widely quoted 1955 paper was called:* Henry K. Beecher, "The Powerful Placebo," *Journal of the American Medical Association* 159:1602–1606, 1955. Another important American advocate for both the importance of randomized controlled trials, and the power of the placebo response, was Harry Gold. See for example the Cornell Conference on Therapy (organized by Gold), "The Use of Placebos in Therapy," *New York Journal of Medicine* 46:1718–1727, 1946.

30 *During the last half-century:* I developed my own view on the ethics of giving placebos, and using the placebo response in treatment, most thoroughly in "The Lie That Heals: The Ethics of Giving Placebos," *Annals of Internal Medicine* 97:112–118, 1982; and later reviewed the topic in "Placebo" in the *Encyclopedia of Bioethics* (2nd edition), edited by Warren T. Reich (New York: Macmillan, 1995), 4:1951–1953. The latter article gives a number of references to other scholarly treatments of the subject. For a more permissive view on prescribing placebos, see among others Howard M. Spiro, *Doctors, Patients, and Placebos* (New Haven: Yale University Press, 1986), pp. 117–134.

30 *The Scottish physician Dr. John Gregory:* A recent, thorough study of Gregory's legacy is Laurence B. McCullough, *John Gregory and the Invention of Professional Medical Ethics and the Profession of Medicine* (Boston: Kluwer Academic Publishers, 1998).

The Placebo Response: Which of Us Is Eligible?

32 *"I regard the placebo response . . . "* Andrew Weil, *Spontaneous Healing* (New York: Fawcett Columbine, 1995), p. 52.

32 *Dueling Acupuncturists:* I owe this anecdote to Daniel Moerman.

33 *[A] nuisance (even if a necessary nuisance) when used:* Patrick D. Wall, "The Placebo Effect: An Unpopular Topic," *Pain* 51:1–3, 1992, is as the title suggests a good review of why the word "placebo" has acquired such a negative connotation in modern medicine and in medical research. Another thoughtful paper on this theme is Nikola Biller, "The Placebo Effect: Mocking or Mirroring Medicine?" *Perspectives in Biology and Medicine* 42:398–401, 1999.

34 *In the 1950s and 1960s, a good deal of attention was devoted:* Typical studies of this sort include Louis Lasagna, Frederick Mosteller, John M. von Felsinger, and Henry K. Beecher, "A Study of the Placebo Response," *American Journal of Medicine* 16:770–779, 1954; James Parkhouse, "Placebo Reactor," *Nature* 199:308, 1963; Joseph H. Campbell and C. Peter Rosenbaum, "Placebo Effect and Symptom Relief in Psychotherapy," *Archives of General Psychiatry* 16:364–368, 1967; Michael M. Nash and Fred M. Zimring, "Prediction of Reaction to Placebo," *Journal of Abnormal Psychology* 74:568–573, 1969; Charles G. Moertel, William F. Taylor, Arthur Roth, and Francis A. J. Tyce, "Who Responds to Sugar Pills?", *Mayo Clinic Proceedings* 51:96–100, 1976; Carol J. Fairchild, A. John Rush, Nishendu Vasavada, Donna E. Giles, and Manoocheher Khatmani, "Which Depressions Respond to Placebo?", *Psychiatry Research* 18:217–226, 1986. Another helpful review is D. R. Doongaji, V. N. Vahia and M.P.E. Bharucha, "On Placebos, Placebo Responses and Placebo Responders. A Review of Psychological, Psychopharmacological and Psychophysiological Factors. II. Psychopharmacological and Psychophysiological Factors." *Journal of Postgraduate Medicine* 24:147–157, 1978.

35 *Clinical Psychologists Seymour Fisher and Roger Greenberg:* Their review of acquiescence as a personality type associated with placebo response is in Seymour Fisher and Roger P. Greenberg, "The Curse of the Placebo: Fanciful Pursuit of a Pure Biological Therapy," in their edited book *From Placebo to Panacea: Putting Psychiatric Drugs to the*

Test (New York: Wiley, 1997), pp. 34–40. An earlier report is Seymour Fisher and Rhoda I. Fisher, "Placebo Response and Acquiescence," *Psychopharmacologia* 4:298–301, 1963.

36 *That acquiescence simultaneously predicts reactions to placebos and active drugs:* This passage is from Seymour Fisher and Roger P. Greenberg, "The Curse of the Placebo: Fanciful Pursuit of a Pure Biological Therapy," in *From Placebo to Panacea: Putting Psychiatric Drugs to the Test,* edited by Seymour Fisher and Roger P. Greenberg (New York: Wiley, 1997), p. 39.

37 *That is, the more anxious the subject:* A good review of studies on this subject is Frederick J. Evans, "The Placebo Response in Pain Reduction," in *Advances in Neurology. Volume 4: Pain,* edited by J. J. Bonica (New York: Raven Press, 1974).

37 *A mythical quest for a "biologically pure" drug:* The quotation is from Seymour Fisher and Roger P. Greenberg, "The Curse of the Placebo: Fanciful Pursuit of a Pure Biological Therapy," in *From Placebo to Panacea: Putting Psychiatric Drugs to the Test,* edited by Seymour Fisher and Roger P. Greenberg (New York: Wiley, 1997), p. 46.

38 *Telling Research Subjects the Truth*: This case study is from Lee C. Park and Lino Covi, "Nonblind Placebo Trial," *Archives of General Psychiatry* 12:336–345, 1965.

41 *People are becoming much more comfortable with the ways the mind and the body can interact:* One of the most prominent advocates for an integration of mind and body in medicine (a biopsychosocial model) was the late George Engel. See especially his essay, "How Long Must Medicine's Science Be Bound by a Seventeenth Century World View?" in *The Task of Medicine: Dialogue at Wickenberg,* edited by Kerr L. White (Menlo Park, CA: Henry J. Kaiser Family Foundation, 1988).

Chapter Four: The Inner Pharmacy

42 *[I] further proclaimed that the body of man was God's drugstore:* Andrew Taylor Still, *Autobiography of A.T. Still* (Kirksville, MO: privately published, 1908), p. 182. I am indebted to Mark Mikols for calling this quote to my attention.

45 *We could think of this set of health-restoring features as the body's inner pharmacy:* This metaphor was first suggested to me by a passage in a thoughtful paper by Roger J. Bulger, "The Demise of the Placebo Effect in the Practice of Scientific Medicine—A Natural Progression or an Undesirable Aberration?" *Transactions of the American Clinical and Climatological Association* 102:285–293, 1990: "It is much easier now to consider the art of medicine as an emerging science through which the adept practitioner allows or facilitates the patient's own internal pharmacy to dispense agents in therapeutic combinations and amounts at just the right time" (p. 290). I did not become aware of the much earlier statement by Andrew Taylor Still until some years later (see above).

47 *There's a popular newspaper cartoon that reads:* The cartoon is "Pot-Shots" by Ashleigh Brilliant. Pot-Shot #5383, Copyright Ashleigh Brilliant, Santa Barbara, CA (http://www.ashleighbrilliant.com).

49 *The fact that individuals can take advantage:* The quote is from Seymour Fisher and Roger P. Greenberg, "The Curse of the Placebo: Fanciful Pursuit of a Pure Biological Therapy," in *From Placebo to Panacea: Putting Psychiatric Drugs to the Test,* edited by Seymour Fisher and Roger P. Greenberg (New York: Wiley, 1997), p. 42.

50 *Drugs for Ulcers: What Dan Moerman Found*: This case study is from Daniel E. Moerman, "General Medical Effectiveness and Human Biology: Placebo Effects in the Treatment of Ulcer Disease," *Medical Anthropology Quarterly* 14(4):3–16, August 1983.

Chapter Five: The Placebo Response and Expectancy

55 *A case was related by the late Dr. Gregory:* "Hahnemannism," *The Lancet,* Volume 1 for 1836–37, p. 374.

55 *Still, physicians and scientists of the modern era:* An excellent review of placebo theories is Connie Peck and Grahame Coleman, "Implications of Placebo Theory for Clinical Research and Practice in Pain Management," *Theoretical Medicine* 12:247–270, 1991.

56 *Now let's look in detail at expectancy:* Some articles on expectancy theory include: Marianne Frankenhaeuser, Birgitta Post, Ragnar

Hagdahl, and Bjoern Wrangsjoe, "Effects of a Depressant Drug as Modified by Experimentally Induced Expectation," *Perceptual and Motor Skills* 18:513–522, 1964; Wallace Wilkins, "Expectancy of Therapeutic Gain: An Empirical and Conceptual Critique," *Journal of Consulting and Clinical Psychology* 40:69–77, 1973; Michael Ross and James M. Olson, "An Expectancy-Attribution Model of the Effects of Placebos," *Psychological Review* 88:408–437, 1981; Mark P. Jensen and Paul Karoly, "Control Theory and Multiple Placebo Effects," *International Journal of Psychiatry in Medicine* 15:137–147, 1985; Irving Kirsch, "Response Expectancy as a Determinant of Experience and Behavior," *American Psychologist* 40:1189–1202, 1985; Frederick J. Evans, "Expectancy, Therapeutic Instructions, and the Placebo Response," in *Placebo: Theory, Research, and Mechanisms,* edited by Leonard White, Bernard Tursky, and Gary E. Schwartz (New York: Guilford Press, 1985), pp. 215–228; Ann B. Flood, Daniel P. Lorence, Jiao Ding, Klim McPherson, and Nicholas A. Black, "The Role of Expectations in Patients' Reports of Post-Operative Outcomes and Improvement Following Therapy," *Medical Care* 31:1043–1056, 1993.

56 *Tom, The Placebo Responder:* Stewart Wolf, "Effects of Suggestion and Conditioning on the Action of Chemical Agents in Human Subjects—The Pharmacology of Placebos," *Journal of Clinical Investigation* 29:100–109, 1950.

58 *Can the Placebo Response Reverse the Chemical Power:* Thomas J. Luparello, Nancy Leist, Cary H. Lourie, and Pauline Sweet, "The Interaction of Psychologic Stimuli and Pharmacologic Agents on Airway Reactivity in Asthmatic Subjects," *Psychosomatic Medicine* 32:509–513, 1970. Later studies on asthma included Carole Butler and Andrew Steptoe, "Placebo Responses: An Experimental Study of Psychophysiological Processes in Asthmatic Volunteers," *British Journal of Clinical Psychology* 25:173–183, 1986; and A.I. Boner, G. Vallone, D.G. Peroni, G.L. Piacentini, and D. Gaburro, "Efficacy and Duration of Action of Placebo Responses in the Prevention of Exercise-Induced Asthma in Children," *Journal of Asthma* 25:1–5, 1988. Richard A. Lewis, Martin N. Lewis, and Anne E. Tattersfield, "Asthma Induced by

Suggestion: Is It Due to Airway Cooling?" *American Review of Respiratory Diseases* 129:691–695, 1984, argued that bronchoconstriction (worsening of asthma) that had been attributed to placebos and suggestion might actually be due to the cooling of the air passages by the mist. This would not explain the findings of some earlier studies, however, and later studies using mist carefully warmed to body temperature found generally the same results. As we will see in chapter 10, even the most severe critics of the placebo literature agree that the findings of placebo responses in asthma are especially striking.

59 *A final experiment of this type:* Yujiro Ikemi and Shunji Nakagawa, "A Psychosomatic Study of Contagious Dermatitis," *Kyoshu Journal of Medical Science* 15:335–350, 1962. This study is summarized by Herbert Benson in his book *Timeless Healing: The Power and Biology of Belief* (with Marg Stark) (New York: Fireside, 1996), pp. 58–59.

59 *One study comparing the effects of chloral hydrate:* S.B. Lyerly, S. Ross, A.D. Krugman, and D. Clyde, "Drugs and Placebos: The Effects of Instruction upon Performance and Mood Under Amphetamine Sulphate and Chloral Hydrate," *Journal of Abnormal and Social Psychology* 68:321–327, 1964.

59 *Surgery for Coronary Disease:* A comprehensive review of the placebo effect in angina is Herbert Benson and David P. McCallie, Jr., "Angina Pectoris and the Placebo Effect," *New England Journal of Medicine* 300:1424–1429, 1979.

61 *Recently, psychologist Alan Roberts and his colleagues:* Alan H. Roberts, Donald G. Kewman, Lisa Mercier, and Mel Hovell, "The Power of Nonspecific Effects in Healing: Implications for Psychosocial and Biological Treatments," *Clinical Psychology Review* 13:375–391, 1993. The reverse effect is also true; a negative or lowered expectancy can detract from the effectiveness of chemically active drugs. A recent study showed that when subjects were given anti-inflammatory drugs for arthritis in randomized double-blind trials, they reported the drugs to be less effective when they knew there was a chance they would receive a placebo than when they knew that the other drug they might receive was another anti-inflammatory medication. On the other hand, they were less likely to report severe side effects when they knew that they might be receiving a placebo: Paula A. Rochon, Malcolm A. Binns, Jason A. Litner, et al., "Are Randomized Controlled Trial Outcomes Influenced by the Inclusion of a Placebo Group? A Systematic Review of Nonsteroidal Antiinflammatory Drug Trials for Arthritis Treatment," *Journal of Clinical Epidemiology* 52:113–122, 1999.

62 *Here again, the benefits those first subjects obtained from the sham surgery:* A classic paper, arguing that the response to placebo cannot easily be distinguished from response to "active" drug, is Louis Lasagna, V.G. Laties, and J.L. Dohan, "Further Studies on the 'Pharmacology' of Placebo Administration," *Journal of Clinical Investigation* 37:533–537, 1958.

62 *Seymour Fisher and Roger Greenberg emphasize this in their review of research:* Seymour Fisher and Roger P. Greenberg, "The Curse of the Placebo: Fanciful Pursuit of a Pure Biological Therapy," in *From Placebo to Panacea: Putting Psychiatric Drugs to the Test,* edited by Seymour Fisher and Roger P. Greenberg (New York: Wiley, 1997), pp. 23–24.

Irving Kirsch and Guy Saperstein approached this question in a slightly different way, using a careful statistical analysis of 19 randomized trials comparing anti-depressants and placebo (much the same way that Dan Moerman studied placebo vs. cimetidine, as we saw in chapter 3). Kirsch and Saperstein argued that approximately 70 percent of the activity of antidepressant medication is due to the placebo response; and they suggested that much of the rest of the effect could be due to the antidepressant functioning as an "active placebo" (i.e., because of the side effects, people know they are getting the real drug and so respond better). Their study, "Listening to Prozac but Hearing Placebo: A Meta-Analysis of Antidepressant Medication," was published in an Internet psychology journal, *Prevention and Treatment*, Volume 1, Article 0002a, June 26, 1998;http://www.journals.apa.org/prevention/volume1/pre0010002a.html . When several psychiatrists criticized their methods, Kirsch and Saperstein did an even more sophisticated analysis of a number of other studies of antidepressants and turned up very similar results. Kirsch reported the findings of this new study in an interview with Martin Enserink, "Can the Placebo Be the Cure?" *Science* 284:238–240, 9 April 1999.

62 *Arthroscopic Expectations:* The results of the pilot study of the first ten subjects was reported by J. Bruce Moseley, Jr., Nelda P. Wray, David Kuykendall, Kelly Willis, and Glenn Landon, "Arthroscopic Treatment of Osteoarthritis of the Knee: A Prospective, Randomized, Placebo-Controlled Trial," *American Journal of Sports Medicine* 24:28–34, 1996. The entire study was designed to enroll two hundred patients and Dr. Moseley reported at a conference that the later results were consistent with the findings in the pilot study.

A major debate erupted in 1999 over another use of sham surgery as a control in a scientific experiment—incisions made in patients scalps and burr holes drilled into their skulls, in the control group in a study of fetal cell brain implants as a treatment for advanced Parkinson's disease. Both the subjects receiving the actual fetal cells and those getting the sham surgery exhibited notable improvement of their Parkinson's symptoms for a six-month period. See for example, Sheryl Gay Stolberg, "Sham Surgery Returns as a Research Tool," *New York Times,* April 25, 1999,WK-3. For the ethical debate over the use of sham surgery as a control, see Thomas B. Freeman, Dorothy E. Vawter, Paul E. Leaverton, *et al.*, "The Use of Placebo Surgery in Controlled Trails of a Cellular-Based Therapy for Parkinson's Disease," *New England Journal of Medicine* 341:988-92, 1999; and Ruth Macklin, "The Ethical Problems with Sham Surgery in Clinical Research," *New England Journal of Medicine* 341:999-96, 1999.

63 *The Drugs and the Doctors' Expectations:* E.H. Uhlenhuth, Arthur Canter, John O. Neustadt, and Henry E. Payson, "The Symptomatic Relief of Anxiety with Meprobamate, Phenobarbital, and Placebo," *American Journal of Psychiatry* 115:905–910, 1959.

64 *One case report showed a small child:* An inadvertent experiment demonstrating the effect of the parents' expectations on an eight-year-old was recounted by John F. McDermott, "A Specific Placebo Effect Encountered in the Use of Dexedrine in a Hyperactive Child," *American Journal of Psychiatry* 121:923–924, 1965.

64 *In one older study, patients improved more on placebos:* A. Baker and J. Thorpe, "Placebo Responses," *Archives of Neurology and Psychiatry* 78:57–60, 1957.

65 *Many investigators have found that capsules tend to work better:* One good summary of early work on the relationship between the form of the placebo drug and the intensity of the response is found in Frederick J. Evans, "The Placebo Response in Pain Reduction," in *Advances in Neurology. Volume 4: Pain,* edited by J. J. Bonica (New York: Raven Press, 1974). A more recent and more sophisticated study, showing that the placebo effect of injections is stronger than that of oral medication, is Anton J.M. de Craen, J.G.P. Tijssen, J. de Gans, and Jos Kleijnen, "Placebo Effect in the Acute Treatment of Migraine: Subcutaneous Placebos Are Better than Oral Placebos," in the doctoral thesis, *Placebos and Placebo Effects in Clinical Trials,* by Ton de Craen (Department of Clinical Epidemiology and Biostatistics, University of Amsterdam, 1998).

65 *When placebos (or drugs, for that matter) are in the form of colored capsules:* On color effects, see Kurt Schapira, H.A. McClelland, N.R. Griffiths, and D.J. Newell, "Study of the Effects of Tablet Colour in the Treatment of Anxiety States," *British Medical Journal* 2:446–449, 1970; Barry Blackwell, Saul S. Bloomfield, and C. Ralph Buncher, "Demonstration to Medical Students of Placebo Responses and Non-Drug Factors," *The Lancet* 1:1279–1282, 1972; and Anton J.M. de Craen, Pieter J. Roos, A. Leonard de Vries, and Jos Kleijnen, "Effect of Colour of Drugs: Systematic Review of Perceived Effect of Drugs and of Their Effectiveness," *British Medical Journal* 313:1624–1626, 1996. In another study, A. Branthwaite and P. Cooper found that tablets marked with a popular brand name were more effective in relieving headache than unmarked tablets, whether the tablets were really "active" drug or placebos: "Analgesic Effects of Branding in Treatment of Headaches," *British Medical Journal* 282:1576–1578, 1981.

65 *One patient, unlike the average person, became 100 percent convinced:* The "green end first" anecdote is repeated in C.R.B. Joyce, "Non-Specific Aspects of Treatment from the Point of View of a Clinical Pharmacologist," in *Non-Specific Aspects of Treatment,* edited by Michael Shepherd and Norman Sartorius (Lewiston, NY: Hans Huber Publishers, 1989), p. 77. Joyce in turn cites G. Claridge, *Drugs and Human Behaviour* (London: Allen Lane, the Penguin Press, 1970), but gives no precise page reference.

65 *The "bottom-up" processing of the incoming information:* This bottom-up, top-down model is described in Herbert Benson (with Marg Stark), *Timeless Healing: The Power and Biology of Belief* (New York: Fireside, 1996), pp. 72–80. It is also employed in Sandra Blakeslee, "Placebos Prove So Powerful Even Experts Are Surprised," *New York Times,* Science section, pp. 1–4, October 13, 1998, from whom I have taken the "snake-stick" example.

66 *Indeed, Dr. Herbert Benson:* In his book *Timeless Healing: The Power and Biology of Belief* (with Marg Stark) (New York: Fireside, 1996), pp.27–38.

68 *Donald Price and Howard Fields, focusing their attention on placebo pain relief:* See their chapter, "The Contribution of Desire and Expectation to Placebo Analgesia: Implications for New Research Strategies," in *The Placebo Effect: An Interdisciplinary Exploration,* edited by Anne Harrington (Cambridge, MA: Harvard University Press, 1997), pp. 117–137.

Chapter Six
Conditioning Theory and the Placebo Response

69 *"[Richard C.] Cabot's remark . . . that babes are not born."* M.B. Clyne. "The Placebo" [letter]. *The Lancet* 265:939–940, 1953.

69 *In this chapter we'll be studying significant scientific work:* An excellent review of some of the earlier work on this subject is Ian Wickramasekera, "A Conditioned Response Model of the Placebo Effect: Predictions from the Model," in *Placebo: Theory, Research, and Mechanisms,* edited by Leonard White, Bernard Tursky, and Gary E. Schwartz (New York: Guilford Press, 1985), pp. 255–287.

71 *The major experiments that stimulated renewed interest:* The first report of this work was Robert Ader and N. Cohen, "Behaviorally Conditioned Immunosuppression," *Psychosomatic Medicine* 37:333–340, 1975. A good summary of the early work is Robert Ader, "Conditioned Immunopharmacological Effects in Animals: Implications for a Conditioning Model of Pharmacotherapy," in *Placebo: Theory, Research, and Mechanisms,* edited by Leonard White, Bernard Tursky, and Gary E. Schwartz (New York: Guilford Press, 1985), pp. 306–323.

72–73 *In one instance, he was able to try out:* Karen Olness and Robert Ader, "Conditioning as an Adjunct in the Pharmacotherapy of Lupus Erythematosus," *Journal of Developmental and Behavioral Pediatrics* 13:124–125, 1992.

73 *The Vanilla Cure:* At this writing this study exists only as an abstract and not as a published paper: Marianella Castes, Miguel Palenque, Pablo Canelones, Isabel Hagel, and Neil Lynch, "Classic Conditioning and Placebo Effects in the Bronchodilator Response of Asthmatic Children." Presented at Research Perspectives in Psychoneuroimmunology VIII, Bristol, England, April 1–4, 1998. The study was noted in Sandra Blakeslee, "Placebos Prove So Powerful Even Experts Are Surprised," *New York Times*, Science section, pp. 1–4, October 13, 1998.

75 *In summarizing his views on the placebo effect:* Robert Ader, "The Role of Conditioning in Pharmacotherapy," in *The Placebo Effect: An Interdisciplinary Exploration,* edited by Anne Harrington (Cambridge, MA: Harvard University Press, 1997), pp. 138–165.

77 *A Pain in the Arm:* Nicholas J. Voudouris, Connie L. Peck, and Grahame Coleman, "Conditioned Response Models of Placebo Phenomena: Further Support," *Pain* 38:109–116, 1989; and Nicholas J. Voudouris, Connie L. Peck, and Grahame Coleman, "The Role of Conditioning and Verbal Expectancy in the Placebo Response," *Pain* 43:121–128, 1990.

79 *Aware of this problem, Guy Montgomery and Dr. Irving Kirsch:* Guy H. Montgomery and Irving Kirsch, "Classical Conditioning and the Placebo Effect," *Pain* 72:107–113, 1997.

80 *We should keep in mind Fisher and Greenberg's warning:* Seymour Fisher and Roger P. Greenberg, "The Curse of the Placebo: Fanciful Pursuit of a Pure Biological Therapy," in *From Placebo to Panacea: Putting Psychiatric Drugs to the Test,* edited by Seymour Fisher and Roger P. Greenberg (New York: Wiley, 1997), p. 27.

Chapter Seven: The Meaning Model

82 *It is not enough [for the physician] to take an adequate history:* M.B. Clyne. "The Placebo" [letter]. *The Lancet* 265:939–940, 1953.

82 *Dr. Henry Beecher and the Wounded Soldiers:* The anecdote of the wounded soldiers is recounted by Frederick J. Evans, "The Power of the Sugar Pill," *Psychology Today* 7 (April 1974):55–59. Beecher's original paper was "Pain in Men Wounded in Battle," *Annals of Surgery* 123:96–105, 1946. See also Henry K. Beecher, "The Subjective Response and Reaction to Sensation," *American Journal of Medicine* 20:107–113, 1956.

82 *You've already read about Dr. Henry Beecher:* As we've already stated, this was Henry K. Beecher, "The Powerful Placebo," *Journal of the American Medical Association* 159:1602–1606, 1955.

84 *One model especially useful:* I first used the title "meaning model" in *Placebos and the Philosophy of Medicine: Clinical, Conceptual, and Ethical Issues* (Chicago: University of Chicago Press, 1980), pp. 115–130. The component ideas of the model were taken from two sources. The elements of explanation and caring were derived from Herbert M. Adler and Van Buren O. Hammett, "The Doctor-Patient Relationship Reconsidered: An Analysis of the Placebo Effect," *Annals of Internal Medicine* 78:595–598, 1973. The mastery-control element was taken from Eric J. Cassell, *The Healer's Art: A New Approach to the Doctor-Patient Relationship* (Philadelphia: J.B. Lippincott, 1976). An excellent account that has most of the same elements as the meaning model, though divided into four categories and nineteen subcategories rather than collected under three major headings, is Dennis H. Novack, "Therapeutic Aspects of the Clinical Encounter," *Journal of General Internal Medicine* 2:346–355, 1987.

85 *"The Placebo Response Without the Placebo":* Lawrence D. Egbert, George E. Battit, Claude E. Welch, and Marshall K. Bartlett, "Reduction of Post-Operative Pain by Encouragement and Instruction of Patients," *New England Journal of Medicine* 270:825–827, 1964.

87 *A prominent psychologist, Jerome Bruner:* In his book, *Actual Minds, Possible Worlds* (Cambridge, MA: Harvard University Press, 1986).

88 *Quite recently, medical investigators have become seriously interested in the stories:* See, for instance, Howard Brody, *Stories of Sickness* (New Haven, CT: Yale University Press, 1987), and Arthur M. Kleinman, *The Illness Narratives: Suffering, Healing, and the Human Condition* (New York: Basic Books, 1988). Kathryn Montgomery Hunter's *Doctors' Stories: The Narrative Structure of Medical Knowledge* (Princeton, NJ: Princeton University Press, 1991), is about the stories told by doctors rather than by patients, but insists nonetheless that stories are essential to the practice of medicine. Since these works there has been a small explosion in books and articles on stories and narratives in medicine and illness. For a good recent overview see *Narrative Based Medicine: Dialogue and Discourse in Clinical Practice,* edited by Trisha Greenhalgh and Brian Hurwitz (London: BMJ Books, 1998).

88 *For instance, physician Eric Cassell and sociologist Arthur Frank both have argued:* Eric J. Cassell, *The Nature of Suffering and the Goals of Medicine* (New York: Oxford University Press, 1991); and Arthur W. Frank, *The Wounded Storyteller: Body, Illness, and Ethics* (Chicago: University of Chicago Press, 1995).

89 *Care and Concern:* Indeed, what I have been calling here the placebo response, Julian Tudor Hart suggests should be renamed "caring effects": "Caring Effects," *The Lancet* 347:1606–1608, 1996.

89 *In some American Indian and African tribal cultures:* I am grateful to Patricia Marshall for a very vivid description of an African bone-throwing ceremony which brought this point home to me.

89 *"I Don't Want to Be Alone":* The Central American study (from Guatemala) is R. Sosa, John H. Kennell, S. Robertson, et al., "The Effect of a Supportive Companion on Perinatal Problems, Length of Labor and Mother-Infant Interaction," *New England Journal of Medicine* 303:597–600, 1980. The later study in the U.S. was John H. Kennell, Marshall H. Klaus, S. McGrath, et al., "Continuous Emotional Support During Labor in a U.S. Hospital," *Journal of the American Medical Association* 285:2197–2201, 1991. For a further analysis of additional doula research, see Marshall Klaus, John Kennell, Gale Berkowitz, and Phyllis Klaus, "Maternal Assistance and Support in Labor: Father, Nurse,

Midwife, or Doula?" *Clinical Consultations in Obstetrics and Gynecology* 4:211–217, 1992.

91 *The Mother Teresa Experiment:* David C. McClelland and Carol Kirshnit, "The Effect of Motivational Arousal Through Films on Salivary Immunoglobulin A," *Psychology and Health* 2:31–52, 1987.

92–93 *In a classic study of heart attack victims in Israel:* Aaron Antonovsky, *Health, Stress, and Coping* (San Francisco: Jossey-Bass, 1980).

93 *Mastery as Healer:* The specific study first referred to here is Sheldon Greenfield, Sherrie Kaplan, and John E. Ware, "Expanding Patient Involvement in Care," *Annals of Internal Medicine* 102–520–528, 1985. Some of their further work is summarized in Sherrie H. Kaplan, Sheldon Greenfield, and John E. Ware, "Assessing the Effects of Physician-Patient Interactions on the Outcomes of Chronic Disease," *Medical Care* 27:S110-S127, 1989. Other studies on control include Kenneth S. Bowers, "Pain, Anxiety, and Perceived Control," *Journal of Consulting and Clinical Psychology* 32:596–602, 1968; Judith Rodin and Ellen J. Langer, "Long-Term Effect of a Control-Relevant Intervention with the Institutionalized Aged," *Journal of Personality and Social Psychology* 35:897–902, 1977; James W. Pennebaker, M. Audrey Burnam, Marc A. Schaeffer, and David C. Harper, "Lack of Control as a Determinant of Perceived Physical Symptoms," *Journal of Personality and Social Psychology* 35:167–174, 1977; Melvin Seeman and Teresa E. Seeman, "Health Behavior and Personal Autonomy: A Longitudinal Study of the Sense of Control in Illness," *Journal of Health and Social Behavior* 24:144–160, 1983; and Gerhard Schüssler, "Coping Strategies and Individual Meanings of Illness," *Social Science and Medicine* 34:427–432, 1992.

Chapter Eight: The Nocebo Effect

96 *A lady, a patient, informed me:* John C. Gunn, *Gunn's New Domestic Physician, or Home Book of Health* (Cincinnati, OH: Moore, Wilstach, Keys, and Company, 1861), p. 25.

97 *Patty's Big Scare*: This story was recounted to me by "Patty" herself, who wishes to remain anonymous.

99 *It seems probable that Patty would have been the victim of what Dr. Andrew Weil calls "medical hexing":* Andrew Weil, *Spontaneous Healing* (New York: Fawcett Columbine, 1995), pp. 61–65.

99 *Dr. Robert Hahn, who has studied the nocebo effect extensively:* See his recent review, Robert A. Hahn, "The Nocebo Phenomenon: Scope and Foundations," in *The Placebo Effect: An Interdisciplinary Exploration,* edited by Anne Harrington (Cambridge, MA: Harvard University Press, 1997), pp. 56–76. See also his *Sickness and Healing: An Anthropological Perspective* (New Haven, CT: Yale University Press, 1995).

100 *Today, the research on voodoo death:* Walter B. Cannon, "Voodoo Death," *American Anthropologist* 44:169–181, 1942. A more recent skeptical article is J. Reid and N. Williams, "Voodoo Death in Arnhem Land: Whose Reality?" *American Anthropologist* 84:121–133, 1984.

100 *While voodoo death was believed to be real:* Two good reviews are George L. Engel, "Sudden and Rapid Death during Psychological Stress: Folklore or Folkwisdom?" *Annals of Internal Medicine* 74:771–782, 1971; and George L. Engel, "Psychologic Stress, Vasodepressor (Vasovagal) Syncope, and Sudden Death," *Annals of Internal Medicine* 89:403–412, 1978.

101 *The East Templeton Toxin:* Gary W. Small and Jonathan F. Borus, "Outbreak of Illness in a School Chorus: Toxic Poisoning or Mass Hysteria?" *New England Journal of Medicine* 308:632–635, 1983.

Chapter Nine
From Meaning to Bodily Change: The Biochemical Pathways

105 *Nobody has yet devised an experiment:* Ashleigh Brilliant, PotShot #3315. Copyright Ashleigh Brilliant, Santa Barbara, CA (http://www.ashleighbrilliant.com).

106 *Let's begin our discussion of the placebo response pathways:* The ideas in this section were influenced by my attendance at the Harvard University conference on placebos, December 1994, whose proceedings were summarized in *The Placebo Effect: An Interdisciplinary Exploration,* edited by Anne Harrington (Cambridge, MA: Harvard University Press, 1997). Especially helpful to me were the comments of two of Dr. Harrington's colleagues, Steven Hyman and Stephen Kosslyn. Two good general reference sources on the relationship of the mind and the body in health and illness are Brent Q. Hafen, Keith J. Karren, Kathryn J. Frandsen, and N. Lee Smith, *Mind/Body Health: The Effects of Attitudes, Emotions, and Relationships* (Boston: Allyn and Bacon, 1996); and *Mind-Body Medicine: How to Use Your Mind for Better Health,* edited by Daniel Goleman and Joel Gurin (Yonkers, NY: Consumer Reports Books, 1993).

107 *Moreover, we should be aware that some critics:* The case that most psychiatric medications have not been proven conclusively to be better than placebos is argued in *From Placebo to Panacea: Putting Psychiatric Drugs to the Test,* edited by Seymour Fisher and Roger P. Greenberg (New York: Wiley, 1997).

109 *These "inside (the body) morphine" substances were named endorphins*: For a general review see Jon Levine, "Pain and Analgesia: The Outlook for More Rational Treatment," *Annals of Internal Medicine* 100:269–276, 1984. Articles can also be found in standard encyclopedias and medical texts.

110 *Drs. Jon Levine, Newton Gordon, and Howard Fields:* Jon D. Levine, Newton C. Gordon, and Howard L. Fields, "The Mechanism of Placebo Analgesia," *The Lancet* 2:654–657, 1978.

112 *This observation cast doubt on the assumption:* On naloxone and endorphins, see Priscilla Grevert and Avram Goldstein, "Placebo Analgesia, Naloxone, and the Role of Endogenous Opioids," in *Placebo: Theory, Research, and Mechanisms,* edited by Leonard White, Bernard Tursky, and Gary E. Schwartz (New York: Guilford Press, 1985), pp. 332–350; and Howard L. Fields and Donald D. Price, "Toward a Neurobiology of Placebo Analgesia," in *The Placebo Effect: An Interdisciplinary Exploration,* edited by Anne Harrington (Cambridge, MA: Harvard University Press, 1997), pp. 93–116.

115 *Drs. Martina Amanzio and Fabrizio Benedetti of Torino, Italy:* Martina Amanzio and Fabrizio Benedetti, "Neuropharmacological

Dissection of Placebo Analgesia: Expectation-Activated Opioid Systems versus Conditioning-Activated Specific Subsystems," *Journal of Neuroscience* 19:484–494, 1999.

115 *The stress pathway is the oldest example:* Some helpful reviews include George P. Chrousos and Philip W. Gold, "The Concepts of Stress and Stress System Disorders," *Journal of the American Medical Association* 267:1244–1252, 1992; Carol J. Wells-Federman, Eileen M. Stuart, John P. Deckro, et al., "The Mind-Body Connection: The Psychophysiology of Many Traditional Nursing Interventions," *Clinical Nurse Specialist* 9:59–66, 1995; and Bruce S. McEwen, "Protective and Damaging Effects of Stress Mediators," *New England Journal of Medicine* 338:171–179, 1998. See also Brent Q. Hafen, Keith J. Karren, Kathryn J. Frandsen, and N. Lee Smith, *Mind/Body Health: The Effects of Attitudes, Emotions, and Relationships* (Boston: Allyn and Bacon, 1996), pp. 41–80; and Kenneth H. Pelletier, "Between Mind and Body: Stress, Emotions, and Health," in *Mind-Body Medicine: How to Use Your Mind for Better Health,* edited by Daniel Goleman and Joel Gurin (Yonkers, NY: Consumer Reports Books, 1993, pp. 19–38).

119 *The opposite reaction, which Dr. Herbert Benson:* Herbert Benson, *The Relaxation Response* (New York: William Morrow, 1975).

120 *Dr. Dean Ornish has also shown us:* Dean Ornish, *Dr. Dean Ornish's Program for Reversing Heart Disease* (New York: Random House, 1990). Technical reports of Ornish's results include Dean M. Ornish, S. E. Brown, Larry W. Scherwitz, et al., "Can Lifestyle Changes Reverse Coronary Atherosclerosis? The Lifestyle Heart Trial." *The Lancet* 236:129–133, 1990; and Dean Ornish, Larry W. Scherwitz, James H. Billins, et al., "Intensive Lifestyle Changes for Reversal of Coronary Heart Disease," *Journal of the American Medical Association* 280:2001–2007, 1998.

120 *Dr. Ornish and other scientists and physicians bear out:* James S. House, Karl R. Landis, and Debra Umberson, "Social Relations and Health," *Science* 241:540–545, 1988. For a summary see Brent Q. Hafen, Keith J. Karren, Kathryn J. Frandsen, and N. Lee Smith, *Mind/Body Health: The Effects of Attitudes, Emotions, and Relationships* (Boston: Allyn and Bacon, 1996), pp. 261–289.

121 *Research has demonstrated that high catecholamine levels in labor:* See for example Ronald E. Myers, "Maternal Psychological Stress and Fetal Asphyxia: A Study in the Monkey," *American Journal of Obstetrics and Gynecology* 122:47–59, 1975; and Regina P. Lederman, Edward Lederman, Bruce A. Work, and Daisy S. McCann, "The Relationship of Maternal Anxiety, Plasma Catecholamines, and Plasma Cortisol to Progress in Labor," *American Journal of Obstetrics and Gynecology* 132:495–500, 1978.

122 *Psychoneuroimmune Pathways:* Reviews include Lawrence T. Vollhardt, "Psychoneuroimmunology: A Literature Review," *American Journal of Orthopsychiatry* 61:35–47, 1991; Steven F. Maier, Linda R. Watkins, and Monika Fleshner, "Psychoneuroimmunology: The Interface Between Behavior, Brain, and Immunity," *American Psychologist* 49:1004–1017; Janice M. Kiecolt-Glaser and Robert Glaser, "Psychoneuroimmunology and Health Consequences: Data and Shared Mechanisms," *Psychosomatic Medicine* 57:269–274, 1995; Robert Ader, Nicholas Cohen, and David Felten, "Psychoneuroimmunology: Interactions between the Nervous System and the Immune System," *The Lancet* 345:99–103, 1995; and *Mind-Body Medicine: A Clinician's Guide to Psychoneuroimmunology,* edited by Alan Watkins (New York: Churchill Livingstone, 1997). See also Brent Q. Hafen, Keith J. Karren, Kathryn J. Frandsen, and N. Lee Smith, *Mind/Body Health: The Effects of Attitudes, Emotions, and Relationships* (Boston: Allyn and Bacon, 1996), pp. 21–39; and Janice H. Kiecolt-Glaser and Robert Glaser, "Mind and Immunity," in *Mind-Body Medicine: How to Use Your Mind for Better Health,* edited by Daniel Goleman and Joel Gurin (Yonkers, NY: Consumer Reports Books, 1993), pp. 39–61. I was assisted in preparing this section by teaching materials provided by my colleague at Michigan State University's College of Human Medicine, Dr. Kathryn Lovell.

122 *The name psychoneuroimmunology first appeared:* The book is *Psychoneuroimmunology,* edited by Robert Ader (New York: Academic Press, 1981).

124 *One experiment showing this may illustrate:* The Newcastle rat study is described in Nicholas R. S. Hall, Maureen O'Grady, and Denis

Calandra, "Transformation of Personality and the Immune System," *Advances* 10(4):7–15, Fall 1994.

124 *Some scientists have suggested that the body might have an ideal level:* Carolyn E. Schwartz, "Introduction: Old Methodological Challenges and New Mind-Body Links in Psychoneuroimmunology," *Advances* 10(4):4–7, Fall 1994.

125 *Dr. Fawzy Fawzy and his colleagues at UCLA:* Fawzy I. Fawzy, Norman Cousins, Nancy W. Fawzy, et al., "A Structured Psychiatric Intervention for Cancer Patients: I. Changes Over Time in Methods of Coping and Affective Disturbance," *Archives of General Psychiatry* 47:720–725, 1990; Fawzy I. Fawzy, Margaret E. Kemeny, Nancy W. Fawzy, et al., "A Structured Psychiatric Intervention for Cancer Patients: II. Changes Over Time in Immunologic Measures," *Archives of General Psychiatry* 47:729–735, 1990.

126 *So Dr. Fawzy was very careful to explain:* Fawzy I. Fawzy, "Immune Effects of a Short-Term Intervention for Cancer Patients," *Advances* 10(4):32–33, Fall 1994. See also Fawzy I. Fawzy, Nancy M. Fawzy, Lisa Arndt, and Robert O. Pasnau, "Critical Review of Psychosocial Interventions in Cancer Care," *Archives of General Psychiatry* 52:100–113, 1995.

127 *Though research into the placebo response:* For some comments on future imaging studies see Sandra Blakeslee, "Placebos Prove So Powerful Even Experts Are Surprised," *New York Times*, Science section, pp. 1–4, October 13, 1998. I am indebted to Donald D. Price and Laura Symonds for further discussion of these ideas.

Chapter Ten: The Placebo Response and Its Mimics

130 *If you take three groups:* Dr. DuBois's comments were quoted in Harold G. Wolff et al., "Conferences on Therapy: The Use of Placebos in Therapy," *New York State Journal of Medicine* 46:1718–1727, 1946; quote p. 1719.

132 *Still, a small number of critics have argued:* I have already noted that Howard M. Spiro, *Doctors, Patients, and Placebos* (New Haven: Yale

University Press, 1986), is a partially dismissive treatment of the placebo response. Spiro claimed that placebos were largely powerless to change bodily states and could only change the patient's subjective impression (which he nevertheless felt was very important). Other articles expressing skepticism about the extent of the placebo response, or pointing out how other phenomena have been confused with it, include Brian A. Gould, Stewart Mann, Anthony B. Davies, et al., "Does Placebo Lower Blood Pressure?" *The Lancet* ii:1377–1381, 1981; Clement J. McDonald, Steven A. Mazzuca, and George P. McCabe, "How Much of the Placebo 'Effect' Is Really Statistical Regression?" *Statistics in Medicine* 2:417–427, 1983; and E. Ernst and K.L. Resch, "Concept of True and Perceived Placebo Effects," *British Medical Journal* 311:551–553, 1995.

132 *Drs. Gunver Kienle and Helmut Kiene:* "Placebo Effect and Placebo Concept: A Critical Methodological and Conceptual Analysis of Reports on the Magnitude of the Placebo Effect," *Alternative Therapies* 2(6):39–54, November 1996.

132 *We know that Dr. Henry Beecher's 1955 paper:* This, of course, is our old friend Henry K. Beecher, "The Powerful Placebo," *Journal of the American Medical Association* 159:1602–1606, 1955.

134 *Some experts have even stated:* Advocates of a four-armed design include Sherman Ross and L.W. Buckalew, "Placebo Agentry: Assessment of Drug and Placebo Effects," in *Placebo: Theory, Research, and Mechanisms,* edited by Leonard White, Bernard Tursky, and Gary E. Schwartz (New York: Guilford Press, 1985), pp. 67–82.

137 *Studies like those of Luparello:* Thomas J. Luparello, Nancy Leist, Cary H. Lourie, and Pauline Sweet, "The Interaction of Psychologic Stimuli and Pharmacologic Agents on Airway Reactivity in Asthmatic Subjects," *Psychosomatic Medicine* 32:509–513, 1970.

138 *One of the most highly skilled meta-analysis groups:* Jos Kleijnen, Anton J. M. de Craen, Jannes van Everdingen, and Leendert Krol, "Placebo Effect in Double-Blind Clinical Trials: A Review of Interactions with Medications," *The Lancet* 344:1347–1349, 1994. These authors carefully extracted from a large body of medical literature the small number of studies conducted with a "balanced placebo design"—

that is, at least two different groups of subjects received a placebo or "non-specific" treatment, but under somewhat different conditions. This group of studies, at a minimum, would show at least that the placebo response is *not* due to the natural history of the illness or statistical regression to the mean. These studies did in fact confirm the presence of a placebo response, and (very important) the fact that this response also interacts with drug effects.

Chapter Eleven
The Inner Pharmacy at the Interface: Conventional and Alternative Medicine

A viewpoint similar to that adopted in this chapter can be found in Walter A. Brown, "The Placebo Effect and the Integration of Alternative Medicine and Conventional Clinical Practice," *The Integrative Medicine Consult,* January 1, 1999, pp. 16–17.

140 *The real issue for conventional medicine:* Frank Davidoff, "Weighing the Alternatives: Lessons from the Paradoxes of Alternative Medicine," *Annals of Internal Medicine* 129:1068–1070, 1998.

140 *In comparing these two approaches to healing:* A comprehensive reference source is *Textbook of Complementary and Alternative Medicine,* edited by Wayne B. Jonas and Jeffrey S. Levin (Baltimore: Williams and Wilkins, 1999).

141 *Therapy That Fits:* The research described in this anecdote was conducted by Jonathan Bolton, a medical student and master's degree candidate in anthropology at Michigan State University, 1990.

142 *Yet we know all too well the long history of hostility:* A good general reference for this aspect of the history of American medicine is Paul Starr, *The Social Transformation of American Medicine* (New York: Basic Books, 1982).

142 *It's no longer unusual to find conventional M.D.'s:* For a recent review see John A. Astin, A. Marie, Kenneth R. Pelletier, et al., "A Review of the Incorporation of Complementary and Alternative Medicine by

Mainstream Physicians," *Archives of Internal Medicine* 158:2303–2310, 1998.

142 *Once this communication has occurred:* Recently, several major medical journals have signaled the increased interest in alternative medicine by devoting all, or large portions, of one issue to this topic. The editorial comment, however, does not necessarily suggest any softening of traditional attitudes. See, for instance, Marcia Angell and Jerome P. Kassirer, "Alternative Medicine—The Risks of Untested and Unregulated Remedies," *New England Journal of Medicine* 339:839–841, 1998; and Phil B. Fontanarosa and George D. Lundberg, "Alternative Medicine Meets Science," *Journal of the American Medical Association* 280:1618–1619, 1998.

143 *In fact, Dr. Andrew Weil, always a prominent advocate:* See for example Andrew Weil, *Spontaneous Healing* (New York: Fawcett Columbine, 1995). For a more negative portrayal of Dr. Weil's work by the former editor of the *New England Journal of Medicine*, see Arnold S. Relman, "A Trip to Stonesville," *The New Republic,* December 14, 1998.

143 *The appeal of Dr. Weil's open-minded approach:* For a recent account of "integrative medicine" efforts within conventional medical centers, see Leslie Berger, "A Therapy Gains Ground in Hospitals: Meditation," *New York Times,* science/health section, November 23, 1999.

144 *That amounts to saying that conventional medicine:* Mark D. Sullivan, "Placebo Controls and Epistemic Control in Orthodox Medicine," *Journal of Medicine and Philosophy* 18:213–231, 1993.

145 *In a very thoughtful paper, Drs. Ted Kaptchuk and David Eisenberg:* Ted J. Kaptchuk and David M. Eisenberg, "The Persuasive Appeal of Alternative Medicine," *Annals of Internal Medicine* 129:1061–1065, 1998.

150 *One of the first large studies to try to discover:* David M. Eisenberg, Ronald C. Kessler, Cindy Foster, et al. "Unconventional Medicine in the United States: Prevalence, Costs, and Patterns of Use." *New England Journal of Medicine* 328:246–252, 1993. The same group later did a follow-up study: David M. Eisenberg, Roger B. Davis, Susan

L. Ettner, et al., "Trends in Alternative Medicine Use in the United States, 1990–1997: Results of a Follow-up National Survey," *Journal of the American Medical Association* 280:1569–1575, 1998.

150 *Dr. John Astin, of Stanford Medical School:* John A. Astin, "Why Patients Use Alternative Medicine: Results of a National Study." *Journal of the American Medical Association* 279:1548–1553, 1998.

151 *Which is the attitude of groups like "Quackwatch":* Their web site is located at http://www.quackwatch.com.

152 *I must now add that the same defects, which the public at large:* For an analysis of lessons that conventional medicine might take from alternative practices—without granting very much to the efficacy of alternative medicine—see Frank Davidoff, "Weighing the Alternatives: Lessons from the Paradoxes of Alternative Medicine," *Annals of Internal Medicine* 129:1068–1070, 1998.

153 *We've now arrived at the point:* You will recall that this book addresses the placebo response, which is not the same thing as the entire field of mind-body medicine. Thus the advice contained in later chapters includes *some* ways, but not *all* the ways in which your mind can help your body to heal and stay healthy. A very useful guide to the entire field of mind-body healing is David S. Sobel and Robert Ornstein, *The Healthy Mind, Healthy Body Handbook* (Los Altos, CA: DRx, 1996).

Chapter Twelve
Clearing a Path for the Inner Pharmacy: Desire and Forgiveness

154 *And to the degree that I can . . . have . . . compassion*: Dean Ornish, *Dr. Dean Ornish's Program for Reversing Heart Disease* (New York: Random House, 1990), p. 219.

154 *While studying the response of wounded soldiers:* You'll recall that the original paper was Henry K. Beecher, "Pain in Men Wounded in Battle," *Annals of Surgery* 123:96–105, 1946.

155 *More recently, as we saw in chapter 5, Donald Price and Howard Fields:* See their chapter, "The Contribution of Desire and Expectation to Placebo Analgesia: Implications for New Research Strategies," in *The Placebo Effect: An Interdisciplinary Exploration,* edited by Anne Harrington (Cambridge, MA: Harvard University Press, 1997), pp. 117–137.

155 *Fighting Against the Medicine*: This case study is recounted in *The Placebo Effect: An Interdisciplinary Exploration,* edited by Anne Harrington (Cambridge, MA: Harvard University Press, 1997), pp. 228–229.

157 *The pitfall I call the "judge and blame" approach:* Marcia Angell, "Disease as a Reflection of the Psyche," *New England Journal of Medicine* 312:1570–1572, 1985, accused some prominent figures in mind-body medicine of perpetuating this error.

160 *Caroline Myss, in her popular book:* Caroline Myss, *Why People Don't Heal and How They Can* (New York: Three Rivers Press, 1997). The quotation that immediately follows is on p. ix.

160 *She reminds us that these rationalized feelings can extend beyond:* Caroline Myss, *Why People Don't Heal and How They Can* (New York: Three Rivers Press, 1997), pp. 35–36.

160 *Clinging to Illness:* The story of Meg is from Caroline Myss, *Why People Don't Heal and How They Can* (New York: Three Rivers Press, 1997), p. 140.

161 *Ask yourself the question: "What would my life be like:* I learned this question from the family therapy approach of Dr. Janet Christie-Seely. See *Working with the Family in Primary Care: A Systems Approach to Health and Illness,* edited by Janet Christie-Seely (New York: Praeger, 1984).

163 *From Hate to Healing in Oklahoma City:* This story is taken from the newspaper account by Stephanie Salter, "Bomb Victim's Father Heals with McVeighs," *Detroit News,* October 18, 1998, p. 12A.

165 *Scientists are finding that prayer and religious dedication:* Randolph C. Byrd, "Positive Therapeutic Effects of Intercessory Prayer in a Coronary Care Unit Population," *Southern Medical Journal* 81:826–829, 1988; for reviews see Jeffrey S. Levin, "Religion and Health: Is There an Association, Is It Valid, and Is It Causal?" *Social Science and*

Medicine 38:1475–1482, 1994; and Brent Q. Hafen, Keith J. Karren, Kathryn J. Frandsen, and N. Lee Smith, *Mind/Body Health: The Effects of Attitudes, Emotions, and Relationships* (Boston: Allyn and Bacon, 1996), pp. 377–461. However, for a more skeptical assessment, see Richard P. Sloan, E. Bagiella, and T. Powell, "Religion, Spirituality, and Medicine," *The Lancet* 353:664–667, 1999.

166 *Any program of self-healing:* One could be even more general than "forgiveness" and argue that the elimination of rage and hostility should be a part of any self-healing effort. For an interesting case study and review of how anger increases one's risk of almost any disease—and how this risk can be reduced—see Redford B. Williams et al., "A 69-Year-Old Man with Anger and Angina," *Journal of the American Medical Association* 282:763–770, 1999; and for a more technical review see Todd Q. Miller, Timothy W. Smith, Charles W. Turner, Margarita L. Guijarro, and Amanda J. Hallet, "A Meta-Analytic Review of Research on Hostility and Physical Health," *Psychological Bulletin* 119:322–348, 1996. For practical advice on dealing with anger in your life, see the chapter on "Anger" in David S. Sobel and Robert Ornstein, *The Healthy Mind, Healthy Body Handbook* (Los Altos, CA: DRx, 1996).

167 *Sid's Headache:* I heard this story from Dr. Curry at the second Keystone Conference on family medicine, Keystone, Colorado, September, 1988.

170 *Chad's chronic pain:* As a rule, the anecdotes describing patients are taken directly from real cases and are told with only very minor changes to protect each person's privacy. So I need to mention here that "Chad" is a composite case drawn from different individuals and from published case reports.

Chapter Thirteen
Enhancing Meaning Through Stories

174 *I would ask you to remember only this one thing:* Barry Lopez, *Crow and Weasel* (New York: HarperPerennial, 1993).

174 *The next step in harnessing:* We discussed this point at length in chapter 7. Important sources include Jerome Bruner, *Actual Minds, Possible Worlds* (Cambridge, MA: Harvard University Press, 1986); Howard Brody, *Stories of Sickness* (New Haven, CT: Yale University Press, 1987); Arthur M. Kleinman, *The Illness Narratives: Suffering, Healing, and the Human Condition* (New York: Basic Books, 1988); Kathryn Montgomery Hunter, *Doctors' Stories: The Narrative Structure of Medical Knowledge* (Princeton, NJ: Princeton University Press, 1991); and *Narrative Based Medicine: Dialogue and Discourse in Clinical Practice,* edited by Trisha Greenhalgh and Brian Hurwitz (London: BMJ Books, 1998).

176 *What Does It Mean to Break Your Hip?:* Jeffrey M. Borkan, M. Quirk, and M. Sullivan. "Finding Meaning After the Fall: Injury Narratives from Elderly Hip Fracture Patients," *Social Science and Medicine* 33:947–957, 1991.

178 *Arthur Frank, a sociologist who survived both cancer and a heart attack:* Arthur W. Frank, *The Wounded Storyteller: Body, Illness, and Ethics* (Chicago: University of Chicago Press, 1995). Another valuable work by Frank is "Illness As Moral Occasion: Restoring Agency to Ill People," *Health* 1:131–148, 1997.

183 *Mitch Albom's book, Tuesdays with Morrie* (New York: Doubleday, 1997).

190 *Patients who develop this sort of attitude:* It is a sign of our present-day fear and avoidance of death that the very phrase "dying well," once a commonplace idea in the Western culture, may sound to our ears inherently self-contradictory. For an especially effective and moving description of what this means in actual practice, see Ira Byock, *Dying Well* (New York: Riverhead Books, 1997).

Chapter Fourteen
Maintaining Social Connections

192 *The tendency when we're ill is to close ourselves off:* Marc Ian Barasch, *The Healing Path* (New York: Penguin, 1993), p. 345 (quoting Carol Boss).

192 *In a major scientific study widely quoted:* The GUSTO Investigators, "An International Randomized Trial Comparing Four Thrombolytic Strategies for Acute Myocardial Infarction," *New England Journal of Medicine* 329:673–682, 1993.

192 *In fact, these studies show that social isolation:* For an overview, see James S. House, Karl R. Landis, and Debra Umberson, "Social Relations and Health," *Science* 241:540–545, 1988; and Brent Q. Hafen, Keith J. Karren, Kathryn J. Frandsen, and N. Lee Smith, *Mind/Body Health: The Effects of Attitudes, Emotions, and Relationships* (Boston: Allyn and Bacon, 1996), pp. 261–289. Expert statisticians will object that in the text, I have slanted the comparison between the "clot dissolver" data and the social isolation data by quoting the difference in *absolute* risk in the first case (1 percent) and the difference in *relative* risk in the second case (200 to 300 percent). If, however, I had used relative risk in both cases, the 1 percent would have become 16 percent, which still represents a striking contrast.

194 *The good news for animal lovers:* See for example C.N. Wilkes, T.K. Shalko, and M. Trahan, "Pet Rx: Implications for Good Health," *Health Education* 20(2):6–9, April-May 1989.

194 *An inability to make connections may also be due to the fact:* An excellent resource to find out if you may have depression, and not be aware of it, is the patient's guide, "Depression is a Treatable Illness," from the Agency for Health Care Policy and Research (Publication 93–0553), available on the Web at: http://text.nlm.nih.gov/ftrs/pick?collect=ahcpr &dbName=depp&cd=1&t=942848306.

For more on mind-body approaches to managing depression, see David S. Sobel and Robert Ornstein, *The Health Mind, Healthy Body Handbook* (Los Altos, CA: DRx, 1996), pp. 155–165; and Brent Q. Hafen, Keith J. Karren, Kathryn J. Frandsen, and N. Lee Smith, *Mind/Body*

Health: The Effects of Attitudes, Emotions, and Relationships (Boston: Allyn and Bacon, 1996), pp. 215–239.

201 *Granny Q's Kids:* This story was told to me by Arnold Nemore. For more on this and similar studies, see Arnold Nemore, "Seniors Partner with Case Managers on Chronic Care," *Chronic Care Initiatives in HMO's*, Group Health Foundation, March/April 1995. For information e-mail info@ghc.org.

203 *Group Therapy for Metastatic Breast Cancer:* The initial report of the experiment was David Spiegel, Joan R. Bloom, Helena C. Kraemer, and Ellen Gottheil, "Effect of Psychosocial Treatment on Survival of Patients with Metastatic Breast Cancer," *The Lancet* 2:888–891, 1989.

205 *Caroline Myss, reflecting on why:* Caroline Myss, *Why People Don't Heal and How They Can* (New York: Three Rivers Press, 1997); the discussion of "woundology" is on p. 6.

Chapter Fifteen: Taking Charge of Your Own Health

209 *It would be more satisfying to me:* Anatole Broyard, *Intoxicated By My Illness: And Other Writings on Life and Death* (New York, Fawcett Columbine, 1992), pp. 47–48.

210 *Women's Complaints:* Kirsti Malterud, "Key Questions—A Strategy for Modifying Clinical Communication. Transforming Tacit Skills into a Clinical Method." *Scandinavian Journal of Primary Health Care* 12:121–127, 1994.

211 *Remembering to Take Your Placebo Every Day:* The Coronary Drug Project Research Group, "Influence of Adherence to Treatment and Response of Cholesterol on Mortality in the Coronary Drug Project," *New England Journal of Medicine* 303:1038–1041, 1980.

212 *Since that initial study, a number of other large-scale trials:* For a review, see Ralph I. Horwitz and Sarah M. Horwitz, "Adherence to Treatment and Health Outcomes," *Archives of Internal Medicine* 153:1863–1868, 1993.

213 "*To what extent is* my disease *running my life and how much am* I *running my life?*": This question forms a central feature of the counseling approach described by Michael White and David Epston, *Narrative Means to Therapeutic Ends* (New York: Norton, 1990).

218 *Often, the first practical action in managing an aspect:* The idea of breaking a big task down into a number of small tasks is an important aspect of psychotherapy, according to the classic work by Jerome D. Frank, *Persuasion and Healing* (revised edition, Baltimore: Johns Hopkins University Press, 1973). Frank argued that this is one feature that all schools of psychotherapy have in common, and which accounts for much of their success.

223 *Julio's "Faking It":* Caroline Myss, *Why People Don't Heal and How They Can* (New York: Three Rivers Press, 1997); the story of Julio is on p. 151.

Chapter Sixteen
Sustaining a Partnership:
Sharing Control with Physicians and Other Healers

226 *The physician Ralph Bloomfield Bonington is:* The description of the character comes from George Bernard Shaw, *The Doctor's Dilemma* (New York: Penguin, 1954), p. 105. In the Shaw play, it turns out that this character is all placebo and no substance; Sir Ralph is woefully incompetent and knows nothing of the scientific basis for his treatments. But there is no *necessary* reason why having his special personal qualities, which make him a "born healer," need be combined with a lack of scientific expertise. In this chapter I will assume that a solid scientific competence, and the personal qualities that make one a "healing sort of person," go hand in hand.

227 *The Power of Positive Talking:* K. B. Thomas, "General Practice Consultations: Is There Any Point in Being Positive?" *British Medical Journal* 294:1200–1202, 1987. Given my concerns with the ethical use of placebos in practice and research, I must point out a worry that I have with Thomas's otherwise important study— he gives no indication that any sort of consent was obtained from his patient-subjects, or that the study design was reviewed by an ethics committee.

232 *This practitioner seems to regard power:* I discuss the "balance of power" between physician and patient, and the idea that the correct model is a win-win rather than a win-lose model, in *The Healer's Power* (New Haven, CT: Yale University Press, 1992), especially chapters 2–4.

233 *The experience of the late Norman Cousins:* Cousins first reported his experiences to the medical profession in his "Anatomy of an Illness (as Perceived by the Patient)," *New England Journal of Medicine* 295:1458–1463, 1976. Cousins later published a popular book by the same title (New York: Norton, 1979).

236 *Planning Your Visit:* Similar advice to that given below is contained in Tom Ferguson, "Working with Your Doctor," in *Mind-Body Medicine: How to Use Your Mind for Better Health,* edited by Daniel Goleman and Joel Gurin (Yonkers, NY: Consumer Reports Books, 1993), pp. 429–450.

239 *In current medical journals, you can find articles:* The paper I will be referring to most in this section is Nancy Leopold, James Cooper, and Carolyn Clancy, "Sustained Partnership in Primary Care," *Journal of Family Practice* 42:129–137, 1996. Other articles typical of this general trend include Sherrie H. Kaplan, Sheldon Greenfield, B. Gandek, et al., "Characteristics of Physicians with Participatory Decision-Making Styles," *Annals of Internal Medicine* 124:497–504, 1996; and Sherrie H. Kaplan, B. Gandek, Sheldon Greenfield, et al., "Patient and Visit Characteristics Related to Physicians' Participatory Decision-Making Style," *Medical Care* 33:1176–1187, 1995.

240 *By identifying acquiescence as the one personality variable:* Seymour Fisher and Roger P. Greenberg, "The Curse of the Placebo: Fanciful Pursuit of a Pure Biological Therapy," in *From Placebo to Panacea: Putting Psychiatric Drugs to the Test,* edited by Seymour Fisher and Roger P. Greenberg (New York: Wiley, 1997), pp. 34–40.

240 *They quote, for example, one study of depressed patients:* The study is J. L. Krupnick, S. M. Sotsky, S. Simmens, et al., "The Role of the Therapeutic Alliance in Psychotherapy and Pharmacotherapy Outcome: Findings in the National Institute of Mental Health Treatment of Depression Collaborative Research Program," *Journal of Consulting and Clinical Psychology* 64:532–539, 1996.

242 *Before you get too discouraged:* An intriguing report of an expert group on what health professions education would look like, if sustained partnership were placed at the very center of American medicine, is Carol P. Tresolini and the Pew-Fetzer Task Force, *Health Professions Education and Relationship-Centered Care* (San Francisco: Pew Health Professions Commission, 1994).

Epilogue: The Mystery of Healing

246 *Especially those of heightened expectancy:* Alan H. Roberts, Donald G. Kewman, Lisa Mercier, and Mel Hovell, "The Power of Nonspecific Effects in Healing: Implications for Psychosocial and Biological Treatments," *Clinical Psychology Review* 13:375–391, 1993.

247 *We do not like mysteries:* I learned the distinction between mysteries and puzzles from Arthur W. Frank, *The Wounded Storyteller: Body, Illness, and Ethics* (Chicago: University of Chicago Press, 1995). Frank in turn cites the work of theologian William May, who himself credits the philosopher Gabriel Marcel.

248 *The interpretations of the Job story which I find most compelling:* I rely here especially upon David B. Morris, *The Culture of Pain* (Berkeley: University of California Press, 1991), pp. 138–151.

250 *Caroline Myss wrote:* Caroline Myss, *Why People Don't Heal and How They Can* (New York: Three Rivers Press, 1997), p. x.

253 *If we are suffering from an illness right now:* Arthur W. Frank, *The Wounded Storyteller: Body, Illness, and Ethics* (Chicago: University of Chicago Press, 1995). Frank has adopted this phrase from Anatole Broyard, *Intoxicated By My Illness, and Other Writings on Life and Death,* edited by Alexandra Broyard (New York: Clarkson N. Potter, 1992).

253 *Carl Jung is said to have written:* The quote is from Howard Sasportas, *The Gods of Change: Pain, Crisis, and the Transits of Uranus, Neptune, and Pluto* (London: Arkana, 1989), p. 3. I have been unable to locate the work of Jung's in which this appeared.

253 *And in the words of poet, playwright, and president:* Václav Havel, *Disturbing the Peace: A Conversation with Karel Hvizdala,* translated by Paul Wilson (New York: Knopf, 1990).

Index